The Death Of Dieting: Los[illegible]
and Feed Your Body Wh[illegible]

****

ISBN: ISBN-10: 0-9985906-6-5
ISBN-13: 978-0-9985906-6-0

****

Published by Influential Health Solutions LLC in Boca Raton, FL.

Want Free Books?

I'm giving away three free books if you are interested. Please consider signing up at my website:

http://downloadingdaily.com/books/three-free-books/

Also By Chris

The Everspace: Utilizing the Power Of God and Neuroscience To Create Stillness Within

The Back Pain Bible: A Breakthrough Step-By-Step Self-Treatment Process To End Chronic Pain Forever

Table of Contents

DISCLAIMER

AS ADVANTAGEOUS OF A SOLUTION THIS GUIDE IS FOR NUTRITION YOU FIRST NEED TO KNOW TWO THINGS:

1. I AM NOT A LICENSED NUTRITIONIST
2. NUTRITIONAL KNOWLEDGE IS CONSTANTLY CHANGING

THE AUTHOR HAS WORKED VERY HARD TO BE AS ACCURATEAND AS COMPLETE AS POSSIBLE IN THE CREATION OF THIS BOOK. FUTURE RESEARCH MAY BE RELEASED TO THE TOPIC AT HAND AND MAY ADD TO THE VALIDITY OF THIS BOOK OR SHOW THAT THESE CONCEPTS ARE NO LONGER VALID. IT IS A GOOD PRACTICE TO CHECK UP WITH SCIENTIFIC JOURNALS TO KEEP ABREAST OF THIS RAPIDLY CHANGING INFORMATION.

WHILE ALL ATTEMPTS HAVE BEEN MADE TO CITE AND VERIFY SAID INFORMATION IN THIS BOOK, THE AUTHOR ASSUMES NO RESPONSIBILITY FOR ANY ERRORS, OR CONTRADICTORY INFORMATION DUE TO THE VERY FACT THAT EVERY HUMAN BEING WHILE BEING THE SAME STRUCTURALLY, MAY DIGEST AND USE FOOD DIFFERENTLY. AS OF

THIS PRINTING, ALL OF THE INFORMATION IN THIS BOOK STILL WORKS ON A UNIVERSAL LEVEL.

PLEASE NOTE THAT ANY ADVICE OR GUIDELINES GIVEN HERE ABOUT NUTRITION ARE NOT A SUBSTITUE FOR SOUND MEDICAL ADVICE, NOR CLAIM TO TREAT, PREVENT, OR CURE ANY DISEASE. PLEASE SEE A DOCTOR BEFORE STARTING USING ANY OF THESE GUIDELINES ESPECIALLY IF YOU ARE PREGNANT, NURSING, USING MEDICATIONS, OR HAVE ALLERGIES.

IN CLOSING, YOU ARE USING ALL OF THE INFORMATION IN THIS GUIDE **AT YOUR OWN RISK.** THE AUTHOR WILL NOT BE RESONSIBLE FOR ANY INJURY THAT MAY RESULT FROM FOLLOWING THE ADVICE GIVEN IN THIS BOOK.

Prelude

I wrote and first published this book towards the tail end of owning and operating my CrossFit gym in February of 2016. Here we are a little over a year later and I am already revising my first version. If you never thought nutritional information changed that fast, consider yourself informed! The updates this book is going to contain are very exciting to me for two reasons.

One, like a good researcher/experimenter I have already instituted the changes in my nutrition as well as my athletes and clients and we have all reported the same newfound sense of well-being.

Two, It seems there is no limit to the amount of energy you can gain when you eat the correct foods. As I'm nearing my 40th birthday my ability to exercise is still increasing and it is all because of the principles I lay out in this book.

They say hindsight is 20/20. Never is this truer than anything in the health and wellness field. If I knew what I know now about nutrition back when I was growing up my body, and my health would be drastically different than it is today and I am in the best shape of my life right now!

This edition contains updates on how our mitochondria function to provide us with energy. While most people do not need this for every day information, I found the roll they play in our health fascinating and couldn't resist putting it in. Please pay close attention to the revamped carbohydrate and protein sections. There is alarming new information on lectins, as well as alarming new information on the state of the animals we are eating.

When we become informed we can make better decisions, or at least we will understand why we feel the way we do when we make a bad decision. With the revisions in this new edition you will be armed to the teeth with everything you need to know to take your health to the next level and live life to the fullest!

How to read this book

Reading this book should be fun, easy, informative, eye opening, and practically applicable. It is for everyday people looking to make a significant change to their health, and feelings of well-being. Those close to me say I write like I talk (if you would like me to speak to your corporation, gym, or organization about nutrition do not hesitate to contact me. Contact information to follow) so pretend like words in ALL CAPS and **bold** sentences are me screaming those points at you because they are that important ;).

Foreword

Simply put, The Death of Dieting is the easiest way to lose weight. I'm a 5'7", 51-year old male who has struggled with my weight for the last 10+ years. I've topped out at 210 pounds on several occasions. I've tried everything including "leaning out", but the lowest I could get down to was 185 pounds, and every time I always crept back up into the 200 to 210 pound range.

That all changed when I met Chris Kidawski. Chris and I got to talking and he told me he had the easiest way to lose weight. He said it wasn't a diet, but more of a life change. At the time I started his high-speed fat loss guide, I had tried leaning out and had gotten down to 198 pounds from 210 pounds, but had stalled out for 6 weeks. Chris gave me a list of allowable foods and during the first 5 weeks of my life change, I lost 24 pounds. Using this allowable food list, I reached my goal of 165 pounds, losing 33 pounds during an 11-week period.

I achieved this goal without starving myself and without exercising. I didn't eat salads and chicken for each meal. I didn't drink any funky juices or special shakes. I didn't have to buy any boxed meals or try to sell things to my buddies. In fact, I ate a lot of steak and eggs, and organic vegetables like broccoli and cauliflower. I replaced my breakfasts with the most delicious coffee I've ever tasted. I ate portions as big as I wanted.

If you have tried losing weight without success, then The Death of Dieting is for you. The author explains the why and how of the different foods you should be eating and what foods to avoid. He includes guides for high-speed fat loss, maintenance and also a performance guide. These include allowable food lists and sample daily menus, that make it very simple to know what to eat and when you can eat them. If it is on the list, eat it, enjoy it and watch the pounds drop off.

I have had many of my friends tell me that I look 10 years younger. I feel like I'm 20 years younger. I have so much more energy than I did before. The only bad thing was that I had to replace my clothes...... I went from an extra large to a medium!

The Death of Dieting = my weight loss success

Jonathan Martindale
Sunbury, OH

INTRODUCTION – How this book will help me

"We are so attached to our way of life that we turn down opportunities simply because we don't know what to do with them." **~Paulo Coelho**

You Are Not In Control Of Your Own Behavior

I have really terrible timing. Right before the first edition of this book was set to be published, the World Health Organization released a study claiming that processed red meat causes cancer, and is in the same toxin class as asbestos. As I recommend eating red meat I found myself scrambling to revise sections of my book to put peoples minds at ease and defend my position. Fast forward a little over a year later and as I am set to release this second edition that you are now reading, the American Heart association releases a statement renouncing the saturated fat in coconut oil (I recommend supplementing with a lot of coconut oil) and is now putting forth the claim that vegetable oil is much healthier. This sent the Internet into a frenzy.

In George Orwell's book 1984, he puts forth the notion of "thought crimes" by which you can be arrested for thinking an illegal thought. The government had 4 branches that had special powers to control the people. The ministry of peace, which dealt with war, the ministry of plenty that dealt with rationing and starvation, the ministry of love, which dealt with torture and brainwashing, and the ministry of truth, which dealt with propaganda and lies. It is alarming to say that these contradictory names are also being utilized today.

The Food and Drug Administration approves additives that cause sickness (maybe not now, its possible in 30 years, more on this in a bit), the American Heart Association approves grains and vegetable oil that has been proven beyond a shadow of a doubt to damage your heart, and The Academy of Nutrition and Dietetics charges processed junk food companies, the dairy industry, big soda, and candy bar companies $20,000 to put together a fact sheet on their own product and then allows them to offer "educational" seminars to teach registered dieticians what to say to their clients about why consuming their chemically altered food is good for them (21). People go to dieticians looking to make a life change and instead are sold fact sheets on gum written by the Wrigley "science" institute, or facts on dairy by the American "college" of dairy "medicine." And I'm not making this stuff up; sadly (on their part) there is a paper trail for all of this information.

Take this story for instance. In the 1960's, the Sugar "Research" Foundation paid Harvard (YES, HARVARD) scientists in what todays equivalent would be about $50,000 to point the blame at saturated fat as a marker of heart disease (22). Fat gives food flavor so when you take fat out of foodstuffs you need to replace it with something that will make it palatable. Enter sugar. Imagine for a second how tasty skim milk would be without it's added sugar? It would be chalk water. This is what happens when the food industry is paying to have their own research done. They make money, and their product makes you sick. According to Dr. Lustig, author of *Fat Chance – Beating the Odds Against Sugar, Processed Food, Obesity, And Heart Disease*, a group called ALEC (American Legislative Exchange Council) they pay off 338 out of 535 congress people to keep things the way they are in the food industry. Are you taking notice of the names yet? They sound protective, yet are slowly and methodically doing things in opposition of what they are supposed to protect.

I am convinced that there are two things that control how a human develops. The first is how much pain they have encountered in their life, and the second is the food you eat. Both of these factors control your thoughts and emotions, which either spiral you more and more into depression, or lift you up out of it. Food, I'm convinced of it, controls a lot of how you think, feel and act, and the companies that make your food know it. Due to this one fact alone that makes you *not in control of your own behavior* unless you are 100% in control of what you eat.

Everywhere you look you're being told what to buy and what is healthy, yet 30% of Americans are still obese. According to data presented by Congress out of those 30% of obese people, 80% are metabolically ill (a fancy shmancy term for the food you are eating is making you sick), which is 57 million people. You can actually look at these people and realize they are sick. What we also find is that out of the 70% of Americans that are not obese, 40 % of them have the same illnesses as the 57 million people who are metabolically ill, they just don't have the accompanied weight gain. The grand total of the population this adds up to is 67 million people, which means there are more healthy looking sick people in the U.S. than obese looking sick people. Over a third of the population in the U.S.A. is sick because of how the companies manufacture lies in to the manufacturing of your food. Why is this not considered to be criminal behavior?

Companies these days are paying real scientists to create studies and doctor (pun intended) data showing the "health" aspects of their product. These companies are not making food to feed you; they are making food to make money, and they're lying to you to do it and government health agencies are helping them by promoting their products also making money in the process. You're being sold a product, not real food. You're exchanging your hard earned money for a skin condition, asthma, and organ failure. The last time I checked there is no granola bar trees, or Oreo cookie fields. Their delicious, don't get me wrong, but that food did not come from the ground, or come from animals that ate stuff growing from the ground; it came from factories. Nowadays the easiest thing we can do to keep excess weight off is ask the question "Is my food real?" before you eat.

And that's how this book is going to help you. It is going to help you discern what food is real and what food is fake. The fact is that things can get pretty tricky out there. Organic can sometimes not be organic. All natural can be anything but natural, and some of the real food such as meat can be fed fake food before you ate it, which in turn means you are then eating the same fakeness.

Pharmaco – what?

Speaking of fake a couple of other well-hidden terms when it comes to nutrition are Pharmacokinetics, and Pharmacodynamics. Pharmacokinetics is what your body does to a drug, and Pharmacodynamics is what a drug does to your body. The FDA is only concerned with Pharmacokinetics because pharmacokinetics measures how toxic a drug is to your body immediately, where pharmacodynamics measures how toxic a drug is to you over time. For instance, put arsenic in your food and you'll die within minutes. That's why we don't have Whoppers with extra arsenic. Tobacco on the other hand was not regulated at first because after you smoked a cigarette you could go on living a normal healthy life for 20 or 30 years. That's where pharmacodynamics comes in. Artificial sweeteners like sucralose, and aspartame have to go through a rigorous pharmacokinetics profile to make sure they can't kill you within a couple minutes, but there's never any testing on the long term effects. This process provides the neigh sayers with all of the ammo they need because there's no proof diet soda is bad for you even though something with caramel coloring, and zero calories that tastes sweet can't be anything but bad.

There was a study done in 2012 with a bunch of Danish people that were split into four groups. Group 1 was given a liter of soda per day to drink, group 2 was given a liter of diet soda per day to drink, group 3 was given a liter of milk per day to drink, and group 4 was given a liter of water per day to drink. The result? Group 1 gained 20 pounds in 6 month's time, group 2 gained 5 pounds (even though there is zero calories in diet soda), group 3 stayed the same and group 4 lost 4 pounds (no surprise). So even though we can't prove artificial sweeteners are bad for you, we know that you can still gain weight as a result of consuming them, yet people keep consuming them.

I see the same contradiction and befuddlement with diet soda creeping into the so-called organic products as well these days. There's a term called green noise in which manufacturers repackage something to look healthy, even though it is the same old junk. Additives such as brown rice syrup, guar gum, and sunflower lecithin are said to be healthier alternatives yet still have a nice healthy chemical sound to them. They are not doing anything to your body right now, but who wants type I guar gum diabetes, or lecethinitis in 30 years? Not me!

Evolution has designed our bodies in an amazing way. When we eat food not designed for our body we get fat, sick, and then die. When we eat food that was designed by nature for our bodies we can eat as much of it as we want and our bodies have a programmed way of either storing it for energy, using it for energy, or excreting it. As a result we stay slim, healthy, and happy because we are stimulating the correct hormones that induce happiness (Serotonin) rather than pleasure (Dopamine).

Neuroendocrinology studies how the brain controls hormones, which in turn end up controlling the brain. It's no surprise that food controls our hormones, which controls our brain, which in turn controls our hormones some more. It's a vicious cycle that looks like this:

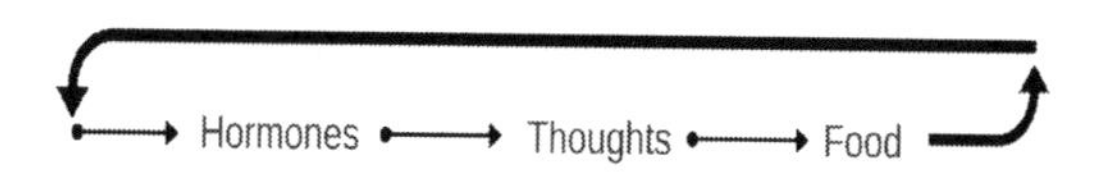

This is where a lot of the dieting confusion takes place because you can actually over consume the wrong type of food on a diet and gain weight, or you can consume too little food and run into a starvation problem, which will not only affect you physically by draining your energy, but mentally as well. This is probably where the term "Hangry" came from. When you consume the proper type of food and manipulate your hormones in a good way, not only do you lose weight effortlessly, stay satiated and energized for hours, but you also start to think more clearly as well. When you balance your food, you balance your hormones, which balances your emotions, which balances your life. Like I said, the health of the mind, and body starts with food, and this is precisely what this book is designed to do for you.

The information contained in this book has allowed me, my clients, my athletes, and several other people to live a pretty phenomenal life. We enjoy high energy levels without the use of 5-Hour Energy or Monster drinks. Our waistlines are slim without counting calories, or starving ourselves. Our bodies seem to be aging slower than most, and our sleep is better than that of a newborn baby. Even though heart disease runs in my family it seems to have stopped dead in its tracks when you get to me, and no this is not because I exercise, it is because of what I eat, and more importantly what I don't eat. If you think exercise is necessary to lose weight, think again. To quote Dr. Lustig one more time - "There is not one study that demonstrates that exercise alone causes significant weight loss, and a meta-analysis (designed to assess significance over many studies at once) proved it; moderate exercise resulted in a weight loss of 2.2 pounds and vigorous exercise in a loss of 3.5 pounds." This shows that the only thing you really have to bust your butt with when it comes to weight loss is what you put in your mouth!

In closing, because I'm sure you're ready to get to the good stuff please remember this. Throughout your daily battles with food I want you to ask yourself this one question before you put anything in your mouth. ***Am I feeding my mind, or am I feeding my body?*** That single sentence ladies and gentlemen will provide more solutions than will ever be found in this book.

CK

For More Information Visit:

http://www.downloadingdaily.com

Or Connect With Chris:

On Twitter: @chriskidawski

On Facebook: facebook.com/chriskidawski

****

While every effort is made to help you learn and apply the information yourself, some people like to go deeper and hire a coach. If you reach the end of this book and still feel dazed and confused, please feel free to contact me for a free consultation. Simply e-mail me at c.kidawski@gmail.com, I read and reply to every email.

****

This book is dedicated to my Mother,

Geraldine Annette Kidawski.

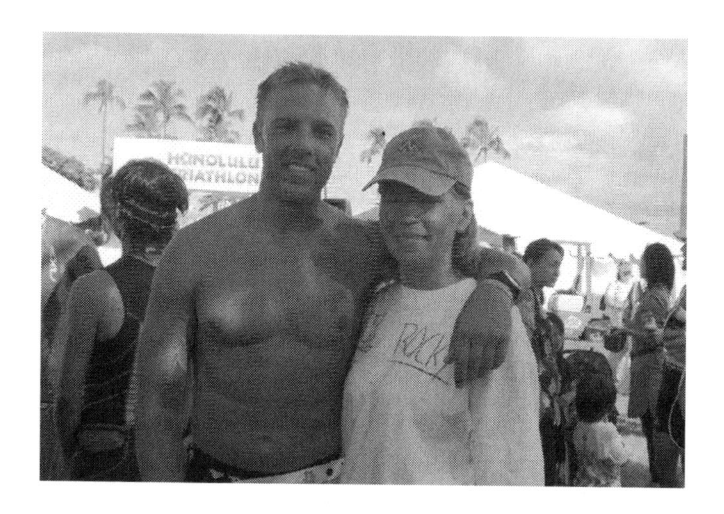

Chapter 1: Fats, But First, Physiology

"The food you eat can be either the safest and most powerful form of medicine, or the slowest form of poison." ~Ann Wigmore

The Rose That Grew From Candy

Derrick Rose was on top of the world as a newly drafted point guard for the Chicago Bulls in 2009. As he began to play he not only dominated other point guards, but almost everyone else as well earning the leagues rookie of the year award in his first season. As Rose played on, his skills developed and so did his trophy stand. He was elected to the NBA all-star team for three straight years from 2010-2012, and was honored as the NBA's most valuable player in 2011. Everything looked hunky dory from the outside, but as a mechanic would say, a different story was brewing under the hood.

Prior to the 2011-2012 season Rose had only missed four games due to a sprained wrist. As the season continued as seasons do, Derrick's "parts" started to "break." A sprained big toe, several back issues, and some odd groin issues sidelined him for 12 games. Twelve shmelve, out of an 81 game season that's not too much to worry about right? Yep. You guessed it. WRONG!

On April 12, 2012 Rose drove the lane with relentless tenacity as only he knows how to do and came to a powerful jump-stop before attempting what looked like a 6-8 ft. shot. As his feet left the floor he haphazardly threw the ball up in the air and grabbed his left knee landing in a considerable amount of pain. Chicago waited with baited breath only to find their mighty domino has fallen with a torn ACL.

Doctors quoted a recovery time of 8-10 months, but Rose was explicit and said he would not return until he felt like he was 110%. Apparently Derrick just wasn't feeling 110% because despite being cleared by the doctors to play, he took the 2012-2013 season off completely. As Rose worked himself into the lineup for the 2013-2014 season, there were flashes of his old self as if nothing happened and everyone seemed to feel relief. But then a hamstring. And then another trip to the surgeon's table with a torn meniscus in the other knee (right).

Rose returned for the 2014-2015 season more determined than ever. After warming up for the first couple of games he scored 32 points against the Washington Wizards on January 14th seeming as if he was on the proverbial "fire." But injury struck again. Was it something new? A shoulder perhaps? Nope. It was the meniscus in his right knee. Again.

Despite losing Rose for much of the season again the Bulls made it to the playoffs that year, losing to the eventual champion Miami Heat. Rose spent the off season healing and came back to the Bulls first practice for the 2015-2016 season healthy as a new born baby only to fracture his left orbital bone. He played 66 games that season mostly with a mask to help the bone heal. He played well, but Chicago was obviously fed up and traded him to the New York Knicks.

Rose's play in New York wasn't bad, but it just wasn't what Rose or his fans were used too. His sharp cuts were gone. His first step looked slow. Rather than darting to the basket he would pull up and opt for a bank shot. Then on April 2, 2017 the all too familiar news came again.

Rose out for the rest of the season with torn meniscus in left knee.

What gives? Is Derrick Rose just injury prone? Is he unlucky? No. I believe he is malnourished.

Mad About Mitochondria

When I was growing up pretending to pay attention in school I can remember being in my first biology class in grade school hearing about the mighty mitochondria. I was around 8 years old and was just introduced to Arnold Schwarzenegger. He was my favorite movie star and I idolized his muscles. I bought a cement weight set from a garage sale for $15 and did nothing but chest and biceps day in and day out. The reason why I remember mitochondria being introduced in grade school is because the teacher called them the "powerhouse" of the cell meaning they were primarily responsible for energy production. I viewed Arnold as a powerhouse, which caused my teachers description to stick in the forefront of my memory still to this day.

Having a masters degree in Kinesiology and being forced to take plenty of physiology classes my knowledge of the development of cellular energy has expanded some and quite frankly the human mitochondria amazes me. Here are some quick facts for you to ponder:

- Researchers estimate that approximately 10% of your bodyweight comes from your mitochondria. Not impressed? 1 billion mitochondria can sit on the head of a pin (17).
- Your mitochondria can produce up to 110 pounds of ATP (the fuel your cells run on) per day.
- Your mitochondria make 10,000 times more energy gram for gram than the sun every second (18).
- Every cell in your heart contains more than 5,000 mitochondria.
- Mitochondrial DNA is passed down only from our mothers. Using specific calculations, scientists have traced everyone's DNA back to one female fossil from 200,000 years ago they affectionately call Mitochondrial Eve.

As I said before mitochondria truly are a powerhouse. But where do they get the fuel to be so powerful? They are fed by the food you eat! Ahhhhh now you see where I'm going with this. The cells that make up all of the structures of our body are replicated using the energy we get from the food we eat. If you replace parts on your car from a junkyard, will you expect them to perform like a new part fresh from the factory?

Of course not.

This leads us into the question, "Do I want my cells to replicate using refined sugars, chemicals, and bleached oils as building blocks?" Or, "Do I want my cells to replicate using grass fed beef, wild caught fish, a ton of fresh vegetables, nuts, and little fruits?"

Probably.

To some people fuel is fuel when it comes to their body. But nobody would use the same gas in a jet as they would in their lawnmower. That would be silly. We need to eat what nature has made for us, not what some chemists concocted during a quarterly board meeting. The food we eat literally makes the contents of our cells, which is called protoplasm. Protoplasm is the living contents of our cells and is where our mitochondria reside. This includes the nucleus and all of the organelles. This is where our cells get their information on how to replicate. If the food we eat doesn't send the right signal, or worse yet no signal at all, then the contents of our cells that make up the structure of our bones, ligaments, tendons, and muscles will not function properly, and we will also lack the proper energy to do basic human tasks like walk to the mailbox or up a flight of stairs. I hope with this detailed information you're getting a picture of just how deep our nutrition affects how our body feels, how resilient the structures will be because of what we eat, and of course how much energy we will have for specific tasks or different levels of exercise. If that's the case then let's get back to Mr. Rose!

A Curious Case of........Skittles?

Derrick Rose has been a self-proclaimed junk food addict for a very long time now. For instance, in an interview with ESPN in 2010 Derrick told the reporter that after his junk food addiction became public knowledge, skittles contacted him and put a custom made machine in his home. He wasn't proud of it and even admitted it was going to contribute to the problem.

During the NCAA tournament in 2008, teammate Robert Dozier threw Rose under the bus in a quick interview when asked why Rose was having stomach issues:

"He just didn't eat - You don't eat and your stomach's supposed to be hurting ... He didn't eat last night or this morning," Dozier said. "We've been having problems with him, making him eat all this year, so it's nothing major to worry about ... He just eats candy and pineapple and syrup. He never really eats real food. Eating grilled cheese sandwiches, things kids eat. He's 19, he eats like he's eight ... He needs (a food pyramid). Someone needs to put one up in his room."

In the same article the head coach of The University of Memphis, Roses' alma mater, is stated as saying he has been stuffing pasta down Roses' throat for a couple days. Pasta is sugar. Actually it's worse than sugar, which you will find out.

Derrick Rose has built a skyscraper in quicksand. His efforts to hire a personal chef in 2010 was too little and way too late. His body has been replicating cells for 22 years utilizing nothing but fast food and candy causing his tissue to have the strength and rigidity of paper machè. With the demands a professional athlete puts on his or her body he never stood a chance. Through my 18 years of strength and conditioning coaching I have found that most athletes need to make a major shift in their recovery efforts (food, sleep, stretching etc.) when they reach the age of 24. What was Derrick's age when he first got injured?

24.

In 2014 Travis Cristofferson released a phenomenal book called Tripping Over The Truth: The Metabolic Theory Of Cancer where he talks about poor food choices, failing mitochondria, and warped DNA replication as causes of cancer. Since then, there have been many more books, and studies reinforcing Christofferson's viewpoints. We don't get cancer, we DEVELOP it!

Could this be true for soft-tissue injuries as well? I obviously think so, and I hope with the information I have already presented to you, you are currently thinking about instances in your life where injury has resulted from binging on Halloween candy, or a severe illness has correlated with a weekend that resembled the movie Hangover. The old saying you are what you eat needs to be changed to you BECOME what you eat. The next step in this sayings evolution is unfortunately you become what you eat, eats, but more on that later. For now, let's get to a favorite topic of mine, which are fats!

Fats Got Fingered

Fats are scary! Nobody knew that better than Ancel Keys. In 1951 Keys went to Europe to search for the holy grail of cardiovascular disease and boy did he find it. Being post WWII many parts of Italy were still under heavy famine as they were rebuilding; locals were reduced to eating plain pizza, pasta, some cheeses, olive oil, wine, and very little meat. The wealthy however could afford more meat and when Keys' wife drew blood samples from both populations, she noticed that blood serum cholesterol levels were higher in the wealthier people who ate more meat. This led Keys to believe that meat and fat was the culprit in heart disease and ran back to America ready to parade his findings and parade he did.

Luckily for Keys, President Eisenhower had a massive heart attack in 1955. Paul Dudley White, the presidents personal physician was a friend of Keys and received the following recommendation from him: EAT

LESS SATURATED FAT! The next day White released a statement advising the public to do the same. As Keys' logic started gaining steam he then used connections to join – and influence the American Heart Association. For the American public this was game over. Keys was heralded as a hero for his discovery and was even put on the front cover of Time magazine in 1961wearing a white lab coat with the title, "Twentieth century's most influential nutrition expert (17)."

Gathering data from other countries, Keys published his Seven Countries Study in 1970 showing that the people who lived in the countries that ate less fat (like Japan) subsequently had less heart disease. The study was majorly flawed though as he ignored data that did not coincide with his hypothesis (he noted that the French eat high amounts of saturated fat and had low cardiovascular disease and just dubbed it the "French Paradox" looking no further) and his findings only showed association, not a link to causation. It didn't matter though as it was the final nail in the coffin for saturated fat. The American public was soon trading in their lard, butter, and bacon for margarine, pasta, and bleached, chemically processed vegetable oil. This shift, coinciding with George McGovern's new grain heavy food pyramid (which we will learn about soon) released in 1977 has spelled big trouble for us ever since.

A recent analysis of our ancestral diet (what we ate during 99.9% of our evolution) suggests a much higher fat intake and much lower daily carbohydrate intake. Think about it, how many cave paintings have been discovered showing gathered berries and nuts? Exact numbers vary depending on what assumptions you use, but carbohydrate intakes of 20-40% (most of which came from low sugar, high fiber vegetables and very little fruits; grains were almost non-existent), fat intakes of 28-60% (which had a significantly different quality than our current diet), and protein intakes of 19-35% of total calories are the current best estimates.

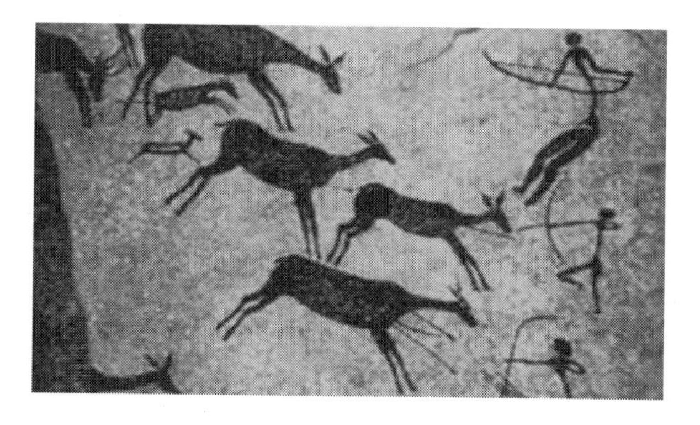

Why did our ancestors not paint pictures of foraging berries?

In our ancestral diet, fiber intakes were monstrous, averaging 100-150 grams per day (currently we get between 8-15 grams per day, 30 is recommended by the FDA). As well, despite the high fat intake, the source of that fat was far, far different than our modern intake. Humans were eating either polyunsaturated, mono-unsaturated, or saturated fat – there was no such thing as trans fat from your processed muffin. Activity levels were also much higher and people generally stayed pretty lean because they had to walk or run everywhere. Alcohol intake was low or non-existent, as was smoking. Although our ancestors dealt with various stresses, they didn't deal with the kinds of chronic stress that occurs in modern societies. There were no alarm clocks, deadlines, traffic, or nasty divorces. A stressor came along maybe once a week, and then the body had a chance to recoup. Nowadays humans are experiencing stress on an hourly basis, and this stresses out our adrenal glands, muscular system, and for sure our digestive system. Compound that with the stress our cells receive from poorly manufactured food and you have a recipe for disease.

Udo Erasmus says, "There are fats that heal and fats that kill." Much has been said about the fats that kill. They are associated with deaths from cardiovascular disease (43%), cancer (23%), diabetes (2%), and other degenerative diseases that kill 68% of Western populations. Only about 100 years ago (an atom in the evolutionary bucket), this was rare indicating that these deaths are from diseases of lifestyle, not genetics. I regularly call bullshit when my clients tell me they have a genetic disease because I was able to lower my own blood pressure using nutrition alone even though heart disease allegedly "Ran in my family."

What lifestyle is creating disease you ask? I'm talking about the up at 5 am, breakfast on the go, 6 cups of coffee, pizza for lunch, then heating up a frozen dinner in the microwave because its "easy" lifestyle. Some people aren't that bad. Some people really try, but the information in the magazines and Internet are so misleading they fail in a matter of weeks to lose even a pound. No amount of trying, or willpower will allow you to lose weight with poor nutrition; it's biologically impossible. Curbing your cravings means controlling your hormones which bad fats and sugars do a really lousy job of. To lose weight, and lose it quickly we need to talk about the good and bad fats, the different types of each, and the ratios that will give us the biggest bang for our buck. Take a deep breath and relax for me – it's not as complicated as you think!

The Bad Fats

I know this may sound like a generalization, but there are so many bad fats jumping off the shelves in our supermarket today that I don't know how else to say it.

"Any and all cooking oil with the exception of first cold pressed olive oil that was not heated, as well as any fats that come in a box or a bag that do not come from a natural source should NOT be consumed."

Natural means it has to exist in nature, which means it was once living. For example, pork belly may come in a box and is full of fat, but the pig we got it from was once living. The fats in cookies come in a box or bag, but we do not have any cookie trees that occur in nature, so for the most part they would be a no-no.

I say that if you are using canola oil, vegetable oil, or any other generic cooking oil, then you are cooking your health. Heat, light, and oxygen destroy oil, no matter the form, and due to the processing of most bulk oils, it is damaged before it even reaches the your pan. By frying your food with it you damage it further. Manufacturers treat oils pressed from seeds with a corrosive base, corrosive acid, and bleaching clays makes cooking oils. This removes 'minor' ingredients, which have major health benefits, but shorten the shelf stability of the oil. So basically these manufacturers take out what is good for us in the oil, and replace it with chemicals that allow it to sit on the shelf for basically ever. When manufacturers bleach oil it turns rancid and smells really bad. The manufacturers must then deodorize the oil to remove the rancid odor, and this process is carried out at very high temperature. Who wants bleach in their frying pan? NOT ME!

In addition to the removal of beneficial nutrients, 0.5 to 1% of the oil molecules are changed into substances that have never been present in nature, do not fit into the very precise molecular architecture of the human (or animal) body, and therefore have highly toxic effects on life's biochemical processes (read: CANCER). You might think that the percentage of these changed molecules is not high, but given their high toxicity, our daily consumption of such damaged oils, and the actual number of molecules that comprise this damage (0.5 to 1%), you are looking at a very serious concern. The following numbers were taken from Udo Erasmus' Website (www.udoerasmus.com) and paint a pretty ugly picture:

- **The oil in a 32-ounce bottle of cooking oil** (1 quart) weighs about 900 grams. A molecule of oil (called a triglyceride molecule) has a molecular weight of between 800 and 1,000 (let's average that to 900 to make the math easy). The rules of physical chemistry tell us that the molecular weight (900) in grams of a molecule (in this case, 900 grams of oil = triglyceride) (i.e. the 900 grams of oil found in a 32-ounce bottle) contains about 6.02x1023 molecules.

- **That number comes out to** 602,000,000,000,000,000,000,000 molecules (12 zeros make a trillion, and 9 zero's makes a billion, so a bottle of oil contains 602 billion trillion molecules). Of these molecules, if 1% is damaged, it means there are 6 billion trillion damaged molecules. If only 0.5% of them are damaged, the number is (only!) 3 billion trillion molecules. How many bottles of cooking oil used in salads, baked goods, fried foods, and hidden in other consumed items does a person eating a 'normal' diet consume in a lifetime?

- **At a conservative estimate of one tablespoon of oil** (containing 10 billion trillion molecules, with 1% or 100 million trillion damaged ones) per day (consumed in salad dressings, mayonnaise, fried and deep fried foods, and hidden oil in baked and other prepared foods), a 32-ounce bottle would last about 2 months. That's six bottles per year. Fifty years of this consumption is 300 bottles over a lifetime. This is a conservative estimate. Many people use substantially more than that (And we wonder why our health fails as we age).

- **Our body contains about 100 trillion cells.** From one bottle of oil, each of our cells would obtain about 6 billion damaged toxic oil molecules. Each daily tablespoon (1% toxic molecules) would provide 100 million toxic molecules per cell per day.

- **How many toxic oil molecules would that person eat over an entire lifetime?** At our estimate, it would be 1,800 billion (or 1.8 trillion damaged, health-destroying molecules).

Studies with bacteria have shown that only 2 molecules per cell of certain nutrients are needed to turn on a gene to alter cell biochemistry. If genes are this sensitive to nutrient molecules, do you suppose that 100 million toxic molecules beating up each cell could affect your genes and have effects on the health of that cell?

If oil does not say 'unrefined' on its label, it has been processed by the methods described above and should be avoided at all costs. A better practice is to use water in your frying pan instead of oil. To prevent overheating and burning, use a lid so the food remains wet. Then it cannot burn. When we burn our meat we turn the burnt parts into matter our digestive system does not know how to get rid of. These become carcinogens (cancer causing substances). Stir or add water to keep the bottom of the food from burning. If you must use, or like using frying oils for flavor, hard (saturated) fats (ghee, lard, coconut oil, palm oil) are damaged less when used in frying than are the other refined liquid oils (I primarily use grass fed butter and coconut oil).

The bottom line reads that the fat in your Starbucks muffin is going to kill you because of the way it was made and processed, while the fat in your eggs or steak are actually beneficial because we as human beings have evolved eating it so it is recognized by our body as safe. Your body will use what it can, and has the ability to eliminate what it can't. It's that simple.

Good Fats

There are over 50 nutrients the body cannot make that it needs for survival, omega-3 and omega-6 fatty acids are two of them. The problem is our ratio of these nutrients that we consume. It should typically be 1:1, but right now the average American diet is 20:1 omega-6 to omega-3. Our omega-6 fats come from all of our land animals. Beef, chicken, pork, lamb, turkey all has high amounts of omega-6 and-9 fatty acids. Fish and plants are our best sources for omega-3 fatty acids.

Like I said, we are looking for a ratio of 1:1, so my question to you is this: Who do you know that eats as much fish as they do beef, chicken and turkey? Not too many people. We need to be conscious of this! For most people, this does not mean eating more fish, but taking omega 3 supplements, which we will learn about in a second, and you can find in the supplement section of this book later on.

When we balance out our ratio of omega-3 to omega-6 & 9 fatty acids, we improve our ability to produce energy. Essential fatty acids make red blood cells more flexible, which means that they can find their way through capillaries more easily. The result is that tissues and cells receive their supply of nutrients and oxygen more effectively, and stamina therefore increases. According to feedback from peer-reviewed studies, this effect is noticeable within a week, usually within 3 days, of adding 3 tablespoons, or more of an omega-3 rich oil blend. Omega-3's increase brain development and brain function. 60% of the weight of our brain is fat, which makes it the fat-richest organ in our body, and one third of that is omega-3 fatty acids. Balancing out these ratios will then undoubtedly elevate mood, and in plenty of cases even lift depression. We can notice now the negative feedback loop eating poor omega-6 & 9 fatty acids can produce. We gain unwanted weight, we feel sluggish, we get depressed and the foods we eat reinforce that feeling of depression!

Our skin is the largest and probably most neglected organ in our body. The environment every single day abuses it. Omega-3 fatty acids form a barrier in our skin against loss of moisture, protect us from dehydration, and prevent many problems involving histamines, prostaglandins, and inflammation. The barrier function of omega-3's helps prevent dehydration, and the constipation and toxicity caused by it. Do some research, next time you're passing through a fast food restaurant, check the hair, skin, and inflammation of all of the customers. We know frying oil is bad for us, and we know that most people who eat fast food have the undesirable 20:1 ratio we talked about earlier. If you notice, their hair will be dry and brittle looking, the skin will not be clear and shiny, and most of them will either be overweight, or be thin with a bloated belly.

One word that is killing the human diet is "snack." I get asked this question all too often. CK, what can I eat as a snack? My answer is always the same, why didn't you eat enough in your meal so you don't have to snack? When we balance out our essential fatty acids, this helps to reduce cravings that lead to constant snacking, one of the main reasons for people being overweight! They also help prevent addictions to foods, and ease the intensity of symptoms during withdrawal from problem foods. This huge hormone restoring effect is not found in any other nutrient we put in our body. Gone are the 6 meals a day crap plans to "keep insulin steady." Gone is the gut destroying granola bars, or mucus producing yogurt cups. Omega-3 fatty acids even lower high triglycerides by up to 65% more than drugs, without the side effects that you get from something like statin blockers used to lower cholesterol. It's pretty amazing that a fat can help lower the bad fats in our body! Lastly, our immune cells use omega-3's to make oxygen 'bullets' that kill cold, and flu viruses, so this means they boost the strength of the immune system too!

Look, the fact is that I recommend eating meat with every single meal you have. Having steak three times a day will NOT kill you. Dietary fat from meats, nuts, and fish can either be used or eliminated from the body because life has developed a code for us to do that. However, the fat that comes in our refined carbohydrates, or the fast food that we eat, gets stuck in our arteries, and stored in our fat cells because the body has no use for it, and no idea how to eliminate it. If you like steak that much, we just need to take a serving of omega-3 oil with every meal we eat to balance our ratios out. That is the key.

Saturated fats

Yes that's right, saturated fats are under the good fat section! The main source of saturated fat in my nutrition comes from grass fed butter, coconut oil, and red meat. Grass fed butter has a very high amount of butyric acid in it, which lowers blood cholesterol, reduces inflammation (especially in the brain) increases insulin sensitivity, and helps our cells produce energy. It's very stable when using it to cook, and you can also put in your coffee which jump starts your brain and allows your body to continue burning fat through the morning (more in a future chapter). There are three different types of saturated fats we can consume and they are short chain, medium chain, and long chain fatty acids.

- **Short chain** saturated fatty acids make up 10% of the total fats found in butter or milkfat. They are also found in coconut, and palm kernel oils. They are easy to digest and people suffering from liver or digestive ailments should include them in their daily nutrition. Butyric acid helps feed the friendly bacteria in our colon, and Caprylic acid (found in coconut oil) is used to inhibit the growth of yeast and candida in our intestines.

- **Medium chain** saturated fatty acids (also called MCT's) are used by the body to produce energy AND CANNOT BE STORED. We get them from coconut oil and my favorite is XCT oil or Brain Octane from Bulletproof Nutrition. You'll find more on these products in the supplement section.

- **Long chain**-saturated fatty acids are used by our body to produce cell membranes. Every cell in our body is a lipid (fat) bilayer and considering we have 100 trillion cells, which means we definitely need this type of fat in our nutrition! This is where saturated fats get their bad name though because long chain fatty acids make our blood platelets sticky. So if we have poor nutrition and our omega-3 to omega-6 ratio is off, then we get a build up of saturated fat in the body and cardiovascular disease follows. However, if we balance out that ratio like we said early, this will NOT happen.

For that reason alone I do not want you to be afraid of eating saturated fats. Don't be that person, who goes to the store and buys a beautiful grass fed, grass finished steak, only to take it home and cut off all of the fat. It's the balance that makes us healthy or unhealthy, not the fat itself! The primary reason saturated fat gets a bad rap is because all of the refined sugar that people eat (without using any of it for energy) ends up being turned into saturated fat by the body. There are two diets that kill, one of them is high fat and high sugar for the reasons just mentioned and you'll learn about the second shortly. Saturated fat in your processed, store bought muffin should be avoided, but the saturated fat in your meat will lead to better health.

Just as a recap so I can be totally clear, because understanding our good and bad fats is so important for our overall health:

- We want a ratio of 1:1 omega-3 to omega-6, 9 fatty acids in our diet daily.

- Omega-3's come from fish and plant sources, omega-6, 9's come from all of our land animals like chickens, cows, lambs, and pigs.

- Saturated fats from natural sources are not bad for us because the body will either digest and use them for energy, or excrete what it does not need. Saturated fats from unnatural sources like muffins, donuts, cookies, or any processed food source are the real culprit destroying our health.

Cholesterol

But what about cholesterol Chris? I'm really worried about cholesterol too! While studying to become a metabolic typing advisor in 2005, I was speaking with one of the instructors and the topic of cholesterol arose. I didn't understand why cholesterol was good to eat, or more importantly, why we shouldn't even pay attention to how much of it we eat. To help clarify her position, the instructor recommended the book, "The Great Cholesterol Con" by Anthony Colpo. To put it simply, it was like waking up one day and realizing there is no Santa Claus. You feel as though for the last some odd years of your life you were lied to by those who were supposed to be looking out for you when you couldn't look out for yourself. Each chapter in Colpo's book was more shocking than the previous.

The following is a breakdown of what I felt were some of the more "in your face," scientifically backed facts about cholesterol. They prove that the American Heart Association (AHA) and Food and Drug Administration (FDA) don't care about us, and we should never really trust anything they say again. As Colpo says in the last sentence of his epilogue, "An independent, rational mind that is prepared to seek out information first hand is a most powerful asset." In the paragraphs that follow, you must be prepared to use your rational mind.

Section 1 is titled, "Why saturated fat and cholesterol don't cause heart disease."

The first chapter of the book doesn't ease you into this widely accepted idea that cholesterol is bad for you. We have to remember that in any age there were ideas that seemed plausible but just weren't so. Zeus shot lightning bolts at the Greeks when he was angry with them, the Earth was thought to be flat, exercising while pregnant was not good, and space travel was impossible. The latest one—cholesterol causes heart disease. Through sound, scientific research, all of these have since been proven false. This book is packed full of medical studies. Here are just some of those claims found in the first section:

- The only way a product can carry an AHA heart healthy logo is by paying a first year fee of $7,500 and then $4,500 every year after. The product is never researched for its heart healthy benefits.

- The highest concentrations of cholesterol are found in the brain and nervous system. They also make up part of the sarcomeres and t-tubules in our muscles. When we take statin blockers our body actually rejects these parts of its own tissue causing a condition called Rhabdomyolysis, which can lead to kidney failure.

- Our liver "recycles" cholesterol to make bile and certain hormones.

- **Several studies have found that higher cholesterol rates are predictive of increased survival rates in older men and women.**

- There is an eleven percent increase in total mortality and a fourteen percent increase in cardiovascular disease for every one mg/dl reduction in our cholesterol rate.

- **The death rate from violence and suicide is double the national average for those following a low cholesterol diet or taking cholesterol-lowering medication.**

- As cholesterol rates decrease so does our visuomotor speed, or how quickly we react in an emergency situation (25% of the cholesterol in your body is found in your brain).

- One study showed that low cholesterol levels were significantly related to Alzheimer's disease.

- Some Kenyan's consume over three liters of full fat cream and two to five kilograms of fatty beef in a sitting yet enjoy a civilization almost free of heart disease.

- In one study, the consumption of polyunsaturated

vegetable oils increased the incidence of cancer and tumor growth in animals (these are the same vegetable oils we use to cook meals for our families!).

- There are cases showing extreme fatigue, amnesia, nausea, kidney dialysis, and even death associated with taking statins, the preferred cholesterol-lowering drug.

- Cholesterol is used to increase cell integrity. This may be why the body channels cholesterol into atherosclerotic plaques, which are essentially portions of damaged cells. If arteries aren't damaged, cholesterol won't accumulate in them.

- Chicken, pork, and steak (all containing high amounts of natural cholesterol) are the only sources of carnosine, which accelerates wound healing, boosts the immune system, rids the body of toxic metals, and even helps fight cancer.

The bottom line here again is that cholesterol has been pegged as the villain, when in fact it is the superhero. Cholesterol is a huge marker for not only mental health, but hormonal health as well. The lower our cholesterol, the less energy we have, because our main sex hormones (testosterone and estrogen) are made from cholesterol!

If you're familiar with cholesterol then you're probably wondering why there isn't any mention of the acronyms HDL or LDL (high and low density lipoproteins). While western medicine wants to peg HDL the good guys and LDL the villains, in reality your body actually needs both!

HDL is made by your body to gobble up cholesterol in the bloodstream and bring it back to your liver to rid it from the body. This is why HDL is so coveted. If I think high cholesterol is clogging arteries and I find a protein that carries it to the liver from the blood for destruction, then that is my superhero! It's just not that simple though.

LDL is what your liver produces to travel out into your body to be used by your organs and cells. Another surprise is that there are actually four different types of LDL utilized by your body, which the standardized test your doctor gives you cannot differentiate between. There's a big fluffy form called large LDL, and then as many as three increasingly dense forms know as medium, small, and very small (aka VLDL) (16). The big fluffy LDL actually increase according to the more good saturated fat we eat from grass fed beef, or coconut oil.

On the flip side, eating a low fat diet that's high in carbohydrates (sugar) actually increases our VLDL, which is very sticky and has a tendency to thicken our blood causes you guessed it – clogged arteries! Combine this with eating bad saturated fats (processed foods) that also have a tendency to thicken the blood and we have a double threat on our hands. There is no doubt in my mind this is the real cause of heart disease. In a healthy person cholesterol is called upon to repair the artery walls when they are damaged through normal inflammation rates and free radical exposure as is evidenced in a book by world-leading nutraceutical researcher Jon Barron called, *Lessons From Miracle Doctors*:

"Quite simply, it says that since your body produces arterial plaque in response to arterial damage, excessive plaque buildup and the concomitant hardening and narrowing of the arteries is a response to excessive damage to the arterial walls. And why only the arteries and not the veins? Because arterial walls contain significant amounts of muscle tissue that make the arterial wall particularly susceptible to damage, while veins contain much less muscle tissue and are thus less likely to suffer damage."

When you are eating unhealthy amounts of bad fats and sugars this repair mechanism breaks and goes haywire creating an unhealthy atmosphere from which cholesterol can do its job. Abuse any one nutrient and the human body will react negatively. Attack any one nutrient in the body and the same negative result will follow. Antibiotics harm good cells, and the virus. Chemotherapy kills good cells and cancer. Statins attack your HDL, and LDL, which are your good guys as well as attacking the bad guys. Forcing the body to kill good cholesterol your body needs with medication in order to drive down a global number now seems to be an exercise of futility doesn't it?

***

What do we do then? Where do we go from here? Risking the chance to sound like a broken record, the health of our arteries, heart, brain, and liver reside in our ability to provide the proper ratios of good saturated fats (grass fed beef, coconut oil (I am definitely breaking that record!)) and reducing our overall daily sugar intake. By doing so we increase the livelihood of our HDL and big fluffy LDL and we decrease the medium, small, and very small, which are our bad guys. Only through this targeted approach, through proper nutrition, can we truly balance these levels out and correct the actual problem, rather than treat the symptom.

Client Story: Laura

Laura was born in Minas Gerais, Brazil into what we American's might call poverty. She was fending for herself, and her brother at the age of six while her parents were in the middle of a divorce and working all day. Growing up she never felt like she had enough food on a day to day basis so it came as no surprised that when she immigrated to the United States at the age of 16 she began eating everything in sight. She quickly gained weight even though her job was very labor-intensive cleaning houses. She described to me with great admiration how rich the food in America was to her and it seemed like she developed a bottomless pit for a stomach. She just didn't know when to say when and came to me 30 pounds overweight with high cholesterol and pre-diabetes at the age of 26. Her doctor had given her a typical diet to follow, which consisted of staying away from all red meat, and consuming lots of chicken, fruits, grains and vegetables. She brought the diet sheet in to me and asked if it was ok for her to follow. I advised Laura it was not the most "Optimal" diet and instead gave her one of my allowable food lists.

Laura began cooking with coconut oil, and putting butter in her coffee. She ate red meat for lunch with her favorite vegetables, and consumed fish or lamb again with her favorite vegetables at night. Within a matter of days she reported back to me how much more energy she had and how the weight was already beginning to fall off.

What I did for Laura was not a miracle; it was using science to trick the brain. The primary reason we get addicted to simple carbohydrates (sugar) is because sugar (along with alcohol, drugs, and gambling) causes the brain to release a hormone called dopamine. Most people want to say that dopamine is a reward hormone and they are somewhat correct. Dopamine is actually released in ***anticipation*** *of a reward. If I do drugs, my high is my reward, and if I gamble, dopamine is released when I win because now I have more than I did before. The reward for eating sugar is weight gain and from an evolutionary standpoint this preserves the species in tough times and keeps us alive, so the brain says bring it on!*

What happens when if we never get into starvation mode? Our reward is never fulfilled and becomes moot. We get fat. Sluggish. Our eating habits become a slippery slope on about a 45-degree decline. There's a silver lining though like I said, and all it took was a little trickery replacing one dopamine response with another.

A research study from the Journal of Nutrition in 2009 reported that we get as much of a dopamine response from fat as we do with sugar (19). It is the combination of both that causes us to binge and overeat, precisely the problem Laura was having. All I did was take the sugar away, keeping the fat, which gave her brain the reward it was looking for. Removing sugar and fat like her doctor was looking to do (except for the fruit which is technically worse than candy, but we will get to that in the next chapter) would have been nutritional suicide for Laura. The brain gets what the brain craves; willpower would have futile in its efforts.

Laura went on to crush her goal of losing 30 pounds in a little over two months. She went back to the doctor after three months for a checkup and was given two thumbs up. Cholesterol levels were normal, and her pre-diabetes was gone. As you will find if you keep reading, there's a really hard way to lose weight, and then there's an easy way. I like easy, and I hope you do too!

The best way to do this is by limiting our protein consumption, which you will learn about in the protein section. As Americans we eat far too much protein on a daily basis specifically from poor meat sources, which contains the artery damaging amino acid homocysteine, which leads me to my second point.

We must eat meat that was born, raised, and finished eating an indigenous diet. For cows it's grass, for chicken it's insects, for fish it must be wild caught not farmed which is fed soy. It may taste delicious once seasoned and cooked but it is actually damaged, which leads me to my third point.

Restrict your consumption of omega-6 fatty acids, which create inflammation in the absence of our omega-3's. Omeg-6's come from all of our land animals so eating steak for every meal is out. There must be variety in our nutrition when it comes to fat and protein.

Finally, restrict grain, and sugar consumption especially in combination with a high fat meal. Chicken Parmesan while tasty is a perfect example of this high fat (fried chicken, cheese), high sugar (pasta is all sugar when digested and hits your blood stream like a lightning bolt!) meal we must avoid. Once every 6 weeks won't kill us, but on a daily or even weekly basis it is cause for concern.

Cholesterol is a heavily misunderstood topic and there are enough triple bypass stories out there that can fill volumes of Stephen King novels. I hope this section shed some light on the subject for you and even though my nutritional guides have taken people off of their cholesterol medication, please consult your doctor before stop taking yours. If you do, send me a message at c.kidawski@gmail.com and let me know, I'd love to hear from you!

Nuts

Nuts are a great source of energy. The problem with nuts is that most all manufacturers of nuts roast them before they package them and send them out to the stores. Nuts are primarily made up of fat, which means they contain natural oils in them. Light, heat, and oxygen just like the cooking oils mentioned above damage these natural oils. This is why nature has provided nuts with a shell!

Nuts also have a generous amount of fiber in them as well. Have you ever gone to a bar, or a party and eaten 10 handfuls of peanuts, almonds, cashews, pistachios, etc.? Ever wonder why, if nuts have a lot of fiber, and fat, that it takes so many handfuls to get you full? This is because they are roasted, the oils are damaged, and you are essentially eating an empty product. That's right, that ten handfuls of nuts had zero nutrients in them your body could use!

When we eat nuts we want to eat them raw. This means no roasting, no honey coating, or chocolate dipping. Preferably we want them right out of the shell (check nuts.com) because even if you buy raw nuts in a clear package the light is still attacking the oils in that nut and decreasing their nutritional value. Here is a list of some of the best nuts to eat raw:

- Brazil nuts – one nut provides 100% of our daily selenium needs, which protects the cardiovascular system, and decreases cancer risks. Selenium is scarce in our diet, so this is important.

- Macadamia nuts – excellent source of fat and are very satiating. Difficult to get out of the shell though which discourages the 10 handfuls of them!

- Walnuts – these are also very satiating due to having the highest content of omega-3 fatty acids in the nut family. They also help fight inflammation, having the highest concentration of antioxidants as well.

- Sesame Seeds – help with balance and vision.

- Pine Nuts – great source of fats, really fill you up!

- Pecans – Filled with polyphenols, which promote the growth of good gut bacteria in your small intestine.

Noticeably absent from this list are two of America's favorite nuts, which are cashews and peanuts. Both of these nuts are technically legumes and contain an extremely high amount of lectins (which we will learn about in the next chapter (so much anticipation!!)).

Peanuts contain a fungus called aflatoxin that can be quite poisonous to our cells, and if you dig poison then you'll be happy to know that cashews are actually in the same botanical family as poison ivy. Cashews have also been studied to create ridiculous amounts of inflammation in the body, especially in patients with rheumatoid arthritis (15).

Just so you can get a real world example, I had one of my athletes ask me if nuts are good as a snack. I told her yes, just make sure they are raw and I explained to her what was already stated above. She then utilized our nutritional journal in our gym software and sent this message in her daily entry:

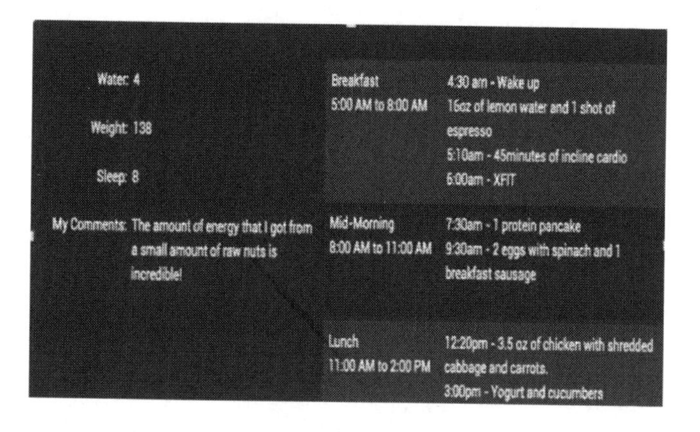

Look at the comments section in the middle left hand side of the picture. This may be shocking to some people but it just shows how powerful of an energy source raw nuts are, and how we take that energy away when we roast them.

If you feel lost without your peanuts or peanut butter I urge you to try coconut butter. It is a truly delicious alternative and is incredibly satiating by providing us once again with our highly coveted omega-3 fatty acids in the form of medium chain triglycerides. Try it and be amazed!

Cheese

Not all cheeses were created equal, I'm sure you know. Cheese can be made from goat milk, sheep's milk, and cow's milk. Cow's milk is the mildest and what most American cheeses are made out of. They are heavily processed and better off in the garbage. I used to eat the Kraft macaroni and cheese by the boxful when I was young just because it was cheap and tasted good. Boy did my stomach get upset from time to time. I'd get colds four times a year and not know why I couldn't stay healthy. I would often eat the Kraft cheese slices as a snack. You'll learn about the health implications of dairy the next chapter, but for now, lets keep our consumption of cow's cheese to a minimum. If you're going to consume cow's cheese, the best come from Europe, so go to the fancy section and choose ones from France or the like. Here are my top picks:

- Camembert – France
- Mozzarella (buffalo mozzarella too!) – Italy
- Emmental – Switzerland (yes, Swiss cheese)

- Taleggio – Italy (smelly, but GOOD!)

Sheep's milk cheese has a little more of a grassy tone, and is a little less creamy than cow's milk, but we don't get the heavy processing of it, and there's no lactose so that is a huge plus for our digestive system. It may be hard to find depending on where you live, but I highly recommend you trying it if you do find it. Here are some for your palate:

- Feta
- Roquefort
- Brebirousse d' Argental
- Abbaye de Belloc
- P'tit Basque

Goat's cheese may sound gross and taste very gamey with a hay/barnyard funk to it, but honestly, some of the best cheese I've had has been an herbal goat cheese. Here are some you may find interesting, or if you want to impress house guests with something different:

- Humboldt Fog
- Garrotxa
- Brunet

- Saint-Maure de Touraine
- Bleu du Bocage

An aggressive estimate would put cheese consumption at about a solid 2-5% of my nutrition. That's it. Even if I eat it alone it's just a slice or two, not the whole block. I'll watch people go overboard at parties tucking the cheese in between crackers, which once again gives us the nasty fat/sugar combo our arteries dread. I'm sorry about that napalm attack coronary artery, but I was at this party and one thing led to another with the cheese and crackers. You understand don't you? No sir, not on my watch or yours. We want the fat only!

That pretty much wraps it up for fats. Knowledge is a great reducer of fear, and now that we are educated about them we don't have to be afraid to eat them. We are turning to carbohydrates next, which in my opinion is a scarier topic than fats, even though they comfort so many people in their time of need. Be prepared to wipe the slate clean on what you think you "know" about the infamous carbohydrate, and ready yourself to get truly educated on this silent killer being promoted as a house pet every day of the week, and twice on Sunday!

Chapter 1 at a Glance:

- The health of your cells resides in how healthy your mitochondria are.
- Light, heat and oxygen destroy oils.
- Vegetable oil, and canola oils are the worst form and should never be consumed.
- Limit fats from sweets,. pastries, and processed foods.
- Balancing out your omega-3 fatty acids to your omega-6 fatty acids will help repair our health.
- Saturated fats are healthy for us and the best types of saturated fats we can consume come from coconut or palm oil.
- Cholesterol is not the devil it is made out to be. Our body needs healthy, natural dietary sources; the liver produces it, and our body also recycles it.
- Low cholesterol levels have been linked to memory problems, depression, and suicide.
- Nuts are best eaten raw and out of the shell as light, heat, and oxygen will harm them.
- Avoid peanuts, and cashews like the plague – they contain powerful toxins!
- Cow cheeses are OK as long as they are from A-2 cows in Europe, or New Zealand.
- Sheep, and goat cheeses are a much better option but should still be slightly limited.

Chapter 2: Carbohydrates

"It is easier to change a man's religion than it is to change his diet" ~Margaret Mead

Zero Is The Loneliest Number?

Out of the three nutrients: fats, carbohydrates, and protein, carbohydrates are the only non-essential nutrient. We can live our whole life without eating carbs. We may not function optimally, look how we want to look, or feel how we want to feel, but we will not die. There are a few tissues such as the renal medulla, red blood cells and the retina that can only use glucose. However, those cells essentially make their own glucose by recycling lactate (produced from glucose metabolism) back into glucose.

The body is able to make as much glucose as the brain and the few other tissues need on a day-to-day basis from other sources. The body is not able to provide sufficient carbohydrate to fuel high intensity exercise such as sprinting or weight training and carbs might be considered essential for individuals who want to do that type of exercise. When carbohydrates are restricted completely, the body still has a small requirement for glucose (although this decreases over time) and the body has to find something to make glucose out of. That something is lactate and pyruvate (produced from glucose metabolism), glycerol (from fat metabolism) and some amino acids.

To be clear right off the bat, I do not recommend a zero carb diet. I did listen to a podcast with a man on it talking about his zero carb diet and even though he experienced good results for himself, he was a physiologist so he understands the restrictions. For the average human reading this book ideally you would want to go no lower than 50, and no higher than 120 grams of carbohydrates per day. This range has been repeatedly shown to produce optimal results for an extended period of time.

For all of you athletes reading this book the body's energy needs for exercise can be calculated quite easily. During weight training, for every 2 work sets (assuming a set length of 30-45 seconds) or so, you'll need 5 grams of carbohydrates to replenish the glycogen used.

So if you did a workout containing 24 work sets, you'd only need about 60 extra grams (24 sets x 5 grams/2 sets = 60 grams) of carbohydrates to replace the glycogen used. So let's say you were starting at the bare minimum of 50 grams per day and were doing roughly 24 sets/workout, you'd need to consume an additional 60 grams (total 110 grams/day) to cover the amount of sugar you burned in energy production. For the average male lifter, this works out to about 1 g/lb. or ~2 g/kg lean body mass carbohydrate per day.

To be clear, if I weigh 180lbs, and have 6% body fat, that means I have 169lbs of lean mass on me, which means I should be consuming 169 grams of carbohydrates a day for full recovery. The problem is that in today's heart healthy grain society, most people have had that much sugar before lunch, and when we consume sugar in the morning (we will go into more detail about this later) our body is programmed to make new fat cells. The only job that a fat cell has is TO GET FULL! So that fat cell starts sending out signals to the brain and we crave more carbs, more quick energy. It's a vicious cycle, and we don't even know it's happening!

The following is a very useful chart taken from the website of world-renowned nutritionist Lyle McDonald (www.bodyrecomposition.com) depicting how many grams of carbohydrates are required per day for various exercises. You can use this as a guide if you would like for your current activity levels, but we will get more into how many carbohydrates you need to eat later in the nutritional guide sections.

Circumstance	Carbohydrate Requirement	Grams for an athlete with 160 lbs. LBM
Physiological Requirement	0 g/day	0 g/day

Practical Minimum to Avoid Muscle Breakdown[2]	50 g/day	50 g/day
Practical Minimum for Individuals Who Function Poorly In Ketosis[3]	100-120 g/day	100-120 g/day
Additional Amount to Sustain Low Intensity Exercise	Minimal approaching zero	Minimal approaching zero
Additional Amount Needed to Sustain Weight	5 g carbs. per 2 work sets[4]	5 g carbs. per 2 work sets[4]
Average Recommendations in Bodybuilding Nutrition	1-3 g/lb.	160-480 g/day

Average Recommendations by Mainstream Nutritionists	2-3 g/lb.	320-480 g/day!!!
Average Intake for Endurance Athletes	2 g/lb.	320 g/day
Recommended Intake for Endurance Athletes	3-4.5 g/lb.	480-720 g/day
Practical Maximum for Non-Carb Loading Individuals	4 g/lb.	640 g/day
Maximal Intakes	~7 g/lb.	1120 g/day

So what are carbohydrates good for then? Carbs boost metabolism, meaning they add fuel to the fire of our engine! Imagine a fire burning kind of slow and then someone throws a balloon filled with gas on the fire.

There will be a bit of an explosion, then the fire will burn hotter, for longer. This is what carbs do when they hit your system.

We mentioned earlier that carbohydrates are not necessary for us to stay alive and that is very true. We will live just fine, however, our performance will suffer. I was on a Ketogenic for a very long time when I was living in Hawai'i. A Ketogenic diet is a diet that relies on solely using fat for fuel. The objective is to stay between 50-100 grams of carbohydrates per day, and no more. This amount of carbohydrates basically goes to fulfilling the basic metabolic needs of the body. What you rely on for energy is all of the fat that you eat. Many people follow this type of diet (The Atkins Diet is a Ketogenic diet) and as long as you are not too active, it definitely works for fat loss and weight loss.

The problem I had was I was working 12 hours a day, and still trying to train for triathlons and marathons, which require a ton of weekly training. I started to lose weight, look almost "skinny fat" and soon could not keep improving my performance. This prompted me to once again research what I was doing wrong and it led me to John Kiefer and his carb-loading theory. What I found out was that for every 4 grams of carbohydrates we consume, the body has to uptake at least one gram of water to assimilate and metabolize the sugar and put it in the muscle cell. My body was essentially "drying" out on the Ketogenic diet. I remember the first night after reading his article I ate and entire mango pie. I woke up the next morning looking leaner and fuller, and I had never slept so soundly in my life. My energy levels were through the roof! But more on this way of eating a little later, the bottom line is that as long as we are eating sugary carbs at the right time, they provide much needed energy for our muscles during exercise. For now, our daily consumption of carbs should be raw, organic vegetables, preferably low on the glycemic index. To somewhat wrap up this introduction on carbohydrates, here are some points worth noting:

- Insulin is released when sugar is present in the blood stream. In the absence of healthy fats the sugar is stored as fat, in the presence of healthy fats, the sugar is used for energy.

- Bad carbs consist of anything in a box or a bag, anything processed, and anything not found in nature (This includes MOST of your beloved healthy all-natural and organic food bars. If you see one of these food bar growing trees or plants in nature please take a picture and I will allow you to eat it. Bottom line is most of them are processed and the manufacturers rename bad ingredients, or create new ingredients that sound organic. What is brown rice syrup anyway?)

- All grains, candies, breads, pastas (especially whole grain pasta!), and fruit (unless in season and grown in your area) should be eliminated or used in moderation or at the right time.

- Fruit: Fruit is as bad as candy. An apple a day will keep the doctor away, but the second will bring you back. Fructose (the main sugar in all fruit) is only used for glycogen restoration in the liver when it becomes depleted. Very few people are ever in this state so usually one piece of fruit a week is good enough. Excess is stored as fat because when we eat fruit there is nothing in our body that tells us we are full so we just keep eating it. Normal sugar sends a signal to our hormones and our brain to stop eating, but with fruit we just grab piece after piece without thinking and this will cause us to overeat and get fat. Scientific studies show fruit was used by our ancestors to fatten up for the coming winter, which means fruit was really just used as a survival tool. Unfortunately, due to the globalization of the food market, we can now get any type of fruit we want any day of the week and any month of the year. This spells bad news for the people who are unaware of these facts. I freak out when I see shopping carts full of yet to be ripe fruit because those people fell into the trap of what the mainstream media has perceived health to be. More on this in the fruit section.

- Studies on artificial sweeteners are showing that it exhibits an insulin response even if there is no real sugar and zero calories are being consumed. Your brain doesn't enjoy the fact that it tasted sweetness but did not get its reward and will cause you to overeat the rest of the day. Eliminating zero calorie sweeteners in any and all products is an absolute must to keep your hormones and blood sugar balanced.

Hyper Palatable and Hyper Rewarding Foods, or Why Carbs make us Fat.

When you eat highly processed foods, they tend to be what are called hyper-palatable and hyper-rewarding. In essence, what happens when you eat these foods, is that your brain becomes over-excited, and it can't "hear" the signals coming from your intestines on how much food you have eaten, which delays the signal telling you enough has been consumed. This leads to over-consumption, addictive-like behaviors, obesity, inflammation, and especially diabetes.

Food products have been specifically engineered to get you to eat a lot of them. There is a "sweetness" factor scientists have found that literally controls the way the brain responds to the food you eat, constantly making it want more. The technical name for it is called the "bliss" point. A gram or two less than the bliss point, and the food is too bitter causing you to not like it, or can't you eat enough of it for sugar to take its effect. A gram or two more than the bliss point, and it's too sweet, becomes over powering, and you stop eating prematurely as well. The problem for food companies is that there is a limit on how much of their product can be purchased; this limit is called the human stomach. The only way to increase sales is to get you to eat more. This is how big companies make their money; they feed your mind with this chemically engineered food, not your body.

Have you ever sat down and tried to see how much Salmon you could consume, or how much celery? You could be fuller than full, yet if I place a tub of your favorite ice cream in front of you, I'm sure you wouldn't have a problem making more room. Now let's say in the middle of eating this bowl of ice cream, I take it away and put more salmon and celery in front of you, how much do you think you could consume? NONE! This is because sugars, salt and fat do not reside in nature together and the combination makes it hyper-palatable (very good tasting), and hyper-rewarding (enhances the pleasure center and releases too much dopamine) to the brain. We have essentially created foods that our brains never evolved to handle, thus willpower goes out the window. They call these types of substances drugs. So when you're full off of your dinner containing salmon and celery, the sweetness factor in the ice cream is just right to where you can keep consuming more, regardless of how full you actually are.

Recipe Time: Mango Tostones!

Ok, ok. So you can't live without your fat, sweet and salty things or you'll simply fade away into the night and wake up a skeleton one day. We certainly don't want that! I know I shunned snacks earlier telling you to simply eat enough at each meal, but there are sometimes where the mood strikes me just right and I indulge in a snack. Mango tostones is one of my favorites and literally costs $5 to make a massive plate:

Materials needed are 2 green as can be plantains (if you do not have plantains in your area use green bananas), 2 green as can be mangos (yes I said GREEN!), your favorite coconut oil to fry with, and Himalayan or Celtic sea salt.

- Cut the plantains or bananas into 1-inch long segments and soak them in water for 5 minutes.

- Heat your skillet with the oil in it and place the plantains or bananas in until both sides are slightly brown.

- Take them out of the skillet and place them on a cutting board. Use a large wooden spoon to now flatten the plantains or bananas.

- Place them back into the skillet for a minute or two cooking them fully now lightly salting them in the process.

- When finished, place the plantains on a plate with a paper towel on it to soak up any excess oil.

- Cut the green mangos and place them in a bowl and when ready to eat, scoop them onto the tostones.

There you have your sweet (mangoes), salty (Himalayan or Celtic salt), and fatty (coconut oil) snack! But what about the plantains or green bananas? Where do those guys fit in? Green plantains and bananas are called resistant starches. Resistant starches is something we are going to learn about a little later on, but I'll give you the good news now so you don't get too anxious! Resistant starches are chock full of sugars that only your good gut bacteria can feed on. The sugar that you eat in green plantains actually cannot be stored as fat instead help your good gut bacteria flourish in order to beat up the bad gut bacteria and banish things like inflammation and excessive gas. Resistant starches are a true life giving food that most of us simply do not eat enough of. With this recipe, you have no excuse!

Ghrelin and Leptin and Why We Don't Get Full

There are two hormones in our body that control hunger. Ghrelin tells us that we are hungry, and Leptin tells us when we are full. Both of these guys are enzyme and sleep activated. Let me explain.

Sleep Activation:

There was a study done on University students measuring how the amount of sleep we get affects Ghrelin and Leptin. When students were told they are going to get 8 hours of sleep, and were then awakened after 8 hours, their Ghrelin levels were low, and their Leptin levels were higher, indicating there is no rush to consume food. However, when the researchers told the students they were only going to get 6 hours of sleep and woke them up after 6 hours, they found Ghrelin levels to be high and Leptin levels to be low. In this instance, the body is trying to stimulate calorie consumption in order to replace the energy we lost from lack of sleep. Interestingly, there was a third test done. This time the researchers told the students they would get 8 hours of sleep yet woke them up after only 6 hours and didn't tell them. The result? Ghrelin levels still high, and Leptin levels still low.

The conclusion here is that in order for us to control our hunger, we need to do more than just watch the amount and types of foods we consume, we need to get to bed on time consistently. If you find yourself eating all the right foods, and exercising to the max, yet the weight still won't fall off, assess how much sleep you are getting and make a change to devote at least 8 hours a night. I know some of you are saying, "yeah right!" but this is science ladies and gentlemen, not hocus-pocus. MAKE IT HAPPEN!

Enzyme Activation:

Enzymes are little rascals (proteins) that act as a catalyst for all sorts of reactions in our body. They fit like a lock and key mechanism and actually accelerate the body's processes for us. It looks like this:

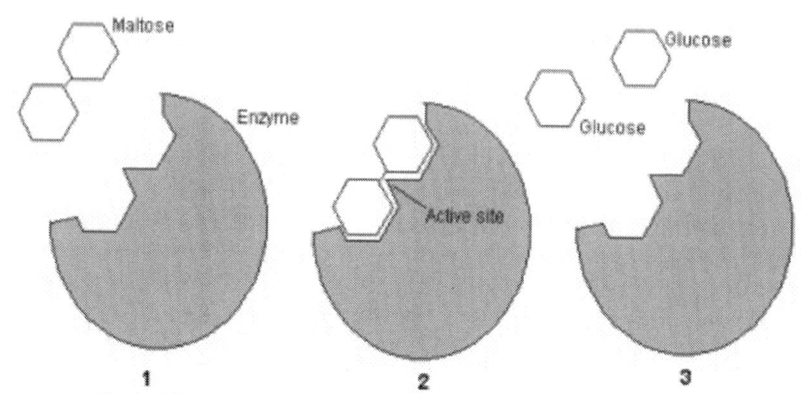

Copied from http://science.howstuffworks.com/life/cellular-microscopic/cell2.htm

The ghrelin activating enzyme ghrelin-O-acyltransferase (GOAT) is present in human plasma and is expressed dependent on body mass index (BMI). Now, even though the BMI is complete crap, what we need to know is that our weight does affect how much of this enzyme we make. Studies show that people with Anorexia, actually make little to none of this enzyme, showing why it is so difficult for people with this disease to consume adequate amounts of food. Their body simply isn't sending a signal to eat! On the opposite end of the spectrum, we have obese individuals. Obese individuals have 34% more GOAT then average weighted individuals, when corrected for weight (3). So not only do overweight individuals have more fat cells sending signals to get full, but they are also making more hormones telling them they are hungry, this is what we call a double-whammy.

Leptin's story is a little bit different. If we are not watching what we eat, Leptin gets tricked most of the time and the brain never gets the signal we are full. The reason for this is because glucose and high fructose corn syrup compete for the same receptors on the enzyme, but only glucose is going to send a signal to the brain you are full. Eating food containing high fructose corn syrup guarantees we overeat because when the key fits into the lock no signal is sent because high fructose corn syrup is literally a chemical concoction that should be avoided under all circumstances.

There was a commercial I saw once where two mothers are talking and a child runs up to one of them asking for a treat. The mom gives him a freeze pop and he runs away happy. The other mother says, "Don't you know that has high fructose corn syrup in it?" The guilty mom says, "Yeah, so?" The other mother says, "Well you know what they say about high fructose corn syrup, don't you?" The guilty mom says, "No, what do they say?" The other mother gets confused and tongue tied and can't seem to spit anything out.

This is the corn industry's way of confusing the public. They are trying to tell us that high fructose corn syrup is ok for us to consume, but the fact of the matter is that it is one of the worst things we can put in our body. High fructose corn syrup has been shown to be one of the reasons there is a rise in childhood diabetes, it has been found to have many toxins in it, including high amounts of mercury, and the worst part is that its 100 times sweeter than real sugar. Companies love it because it costs less to produce more of their product.

As consumers, we get the short end of the stick because we eat double, but our body is only registering single. You see high fructose corn syrup is like paying an employee to come into work, and do nothing. When high fructose molecules attach themselves to enzymes in the body, they stop the enzymes from sending a signal to the brain telling it you are getting enough nutrition and you are full. In return we keep eating more calories to get the same feeling of satiety, and this in turn makes us become overweight. I repeat, avoid high fructose corn syrup at all costs.

Grains

Human beings have been eating food for nearly 3 million years now. Grains popped up about 10,000 years ago but were only sparsely eaten and the actual harvesting of grains started in western Asia, and the Fertile Crescent 3,000 years ago. Grains consist of mainly breads, cereals, pasta, rice, quinoa, tortillas, crackers, chips, grits, noodles, and beans. Grains are advertised as being heart healthy and able to lower cholesterol naturally (remember lower cholesterol numbers actually hinder our health), as well as being a great source of fiber, Vitamin B, iron, magnesium, selenium, and folic acid. The fact of the matter is that these heart healthy grains sitting on our supermarket shelves are just like the oils in clear plastic bottles that destroy our health, except instead of saying refined, they're "enriched."

Enriched is big businesses way of saying, "sorry, we took all the good stuff out, and put just what we think you need back in." They bleach the grains, and then put factory made nutrients back in which studies have shown the body cannot digest and use properly. Congratulations, you just bought edible cardboard. So whom do we have to thank for all of this? Why are grains heralded as the holy grail of health? Because of Senator George McGovern.

In 1977, Senator McGovern appointed a committee of people who knew absolutely nothing about nutrition to devise a nutrition policy titled, "Dietary Goals for the United States." Their primary objective was to cut what they considered to be killer fats, and replace those calories with whole grains. The new policy had five main points:

- Increase carbohydrate consumption to 60% of the diet.

- Reduce fat to 30%.

- Limit cholesterol to 300mg a day.

- Reduce sugar consumption to 40%.

- Reduce salt intake.

Since 1977, obesity, heart disease, hypertension, diabetes, and cancer have all risen. And this isn't even the worst part of it.

Just like animals have teeth to defend themselves, and plants have insecticides to defend themselves, grains have anti-nutrients that bind to nutrients, vitamins, and cellular debris, which then get excreted in our stool so the grain can reproduce. Stated differently, if we eat a large meal containing a significant amount of grains, we can actually have fewer nutrients in our body after we ate the food than before. And I always wondered why I was hungry still and hour after eating a big plate of spaghetti. The grains we know and love today have three main toxins; each one gets nastier as we go along.

Phytic Acid:

Phytic acid is the storage form of phosphorus and is absolutely indigestible. When ingested, phytic acid will bind to calcium, magnesium, zinc, Vitamin B3, and iron and shuttle it out of the body. If it doesn't get excreted from the body, it binds to magnesium and forms crystals that get deposited into the musculature and cause pain. Phytic acid also inhibits several enzymes along the way that are necessary for protein, fat, and carbohydrate metabolism.

Gluten:

Besides gluten giving dough its rubbery feel and ability to rise, there's not much use for it in the body. Before we get to the good stuff, I'd like to tell you an embarrassing story. It was 2006 and I was working in a physical therapy clinic about 32 hours a week. This was a huge shift from the 60-80 hours a week I used to work as a strength coach at the University of Hawai'i. I got bored with all of my free time, so I ended up taking a part-time job as a carpenter on Hickam Air Force Base. Now I'm back up to 48 hours a week working, but the early rising hours began to tire me. I was sleeping on my breaks, I was sleeping before my shifts, and when I got home, I had to take a nap before I did anything. My energy levels were decreasing rapidly and the only excuse offered to me was that I was approaching 30 years of age and this is what getting old feels like. I knew something was wrong though.....

One day I was at the physical therapy clinic and I had just finished lunch about 4 hours ago. It was one of the busiest hours we had in the clinic people were everywhere. As I'm working with someone, I start to get some serious discomfort in my intestines. I start to realize that it's gas so I start to hold it back. Long story short, the gas ended up winning, and kept on winning for about four more hours. I was making everyone in the clinic sick with how horrendous my gas smelled that I had to go out into the alley and continue to relieve myself. It was then that I decided to make a change. As I started to do my research, everything was leading me to gluten being the culprit. As I started to reduce and then eliminate my consumption of grains, and thus gluten as well, my embarrassing problem went away almost overnight.

Gluten has been known to do the following:

- Create an inflammatory reaction in the entire body.

- Cause leaky gut syndrome where pieces of food actually pass through the small intestine undigested and enter the blood stream causing serious food allergies.

- Damage the nerves and the brain.

- Shown to cause seizures, epilepsy, and schizophrenia.

- Can damage the thyroid.

Gluten can be a serious problem for someone who is allergic and should be avoided at all costs. For the rest of us whom get excessive gas it's just an embarrassing issue for us to deal with. I choose not to deal with it. Having a sandwich every blue moon if the mood strikes you will not cause major damage. My main concern is you being educated on what the grains and gluten are doing to your insides. There are other dangers lurking in our grains that we may not want to be so tolerant of.

Chapter 2a: Lectins:

Who Invited You?

Forget that we are talking about grains for a second, and I want you to focus in on the anti-nutrient lectin. Lectins are so dangerous to the human digestive system that they actually deserve a chapter all to themselves. Rather than put them elsewhere I just created a chapter within a chapter! The anti-nutrient lectin is both immunologic (attacks the immune system), and antigenic (can alter the way the immune system functions). It does this by affecting a series of proteins in the body. It has been linked to an increased risk of arthritis, and lupus (an auto-immune disease where the host suffers from fatigue, joint pain, and rashes), and it can damage the cells in our small intestine beyond repair if left unchecked. Lectins can damage our kidneys and pancreas, and has been linked to mitogenesis, or the creation of cancerous cells. Lectins are found in:

- All beans.
- Peanuts and cashews.
- Legumes.
- Cereals.
- Whole grain anything, especially pastas.
- Unripe fruits and vegetables (with the exception of unripe or green plantains, bananas, and mangoes).
- Milk and beef from cows fed grains.

- It can be found in our chicken that is fed a soy or grain diet.

- Farmed fish fed soy and corn.

Lectins are a silent killer and the removal of them from our nutrition really constitutes as a phase II towards achieving greater health. Much of the weight loss people see when they begin my program is due to the removal of processed carbohydrates yes, but it is also from the removal of lectins from their diet!

Whole wheat and whole grain products are extremely addictive. We tolerate the ill effects it produces in our body because we are addicted to them. Most people now know the drug like effect sugar has on our body, and our health, but people have yet to correlate this fact with whole wheat and whole grain foods as well. Like sugar, whole wheat actively promotes weight gain through the lectin wheat germ agglutinin (WGA). It does this in eleven (Yes 11!) ways (15).

1. WGA behaves like insulin which pumps sugar into fat cells not because your body is telling it to, but because WGA is telling it to.

2. It also blocks sugar from getting into the muscle cells where it is most productive and can be used for energy.

3. It interferes with the digestion of protein, and will cause it to be turned in to sugar to be stored.

4. It promotes inflammation by releasing free radicals, which can thin the mucosal lining of our gut (Our small intestine is only one cell thick, but the size of a tennis court, the mucosal lining increase the depth of this barrier for protection).

5. Cross-reacts with other proteins, which creates antibodies that attack our immune system.

6. Crosses the blood-brain barrier taking with it other substances it latched on to, which will cause neurological problems for the host.

7. It kills normal healthy cells.

8. It interferes with the replication of our DNA.

9. It has been shown to cause a hardening of the arteries.

10. It enables the entry of the flu virus by helping it pass through the mucosal lining in our small intestine.

11. Causes inflammation of the kidneys.

Because “whole grains” are so heavily promoted by the American Heart Association, and doctors alike it is very difficult for me to convince people that anything whole grain is destroying their health. It surely was destroying mine, as I once too perceived this to be a “health” food. Lectins are referred to as sticky proteins because they bind to sugar molecules in your system hitching a ride to cause mass destruction. Lectins that are eaten in unripe fruits, vegetables, seeds, grains, rinds, and the leaves of most plants also bind to sialic acid, which is a sugar molecule found in the gut, in the brain, between nerve endings, in joints, all of your bodily fluids, and lastly your blood vessel lining. Using this sugar as a transport there is no area of the body these toxins can’t touch!

This is the paradox we face when eating what we consider to be otherwise healthy plants and vegetables. Surely there’s nothing in a good old-fashioned green pepper that can hurt me, especially if it’s organic! Wrong. The unripe skin is booming with killer lectins chomping at the bit to get past your (laughable) single celled wall of a gut lining. The seeds contain lectins as well and even though red peppers are technically ripe, being in the nightshade family they cause excessive inflammation and consumption must be limited.

The worst part is scientists believe that the rise in Autism actually correlates with the rise in grain consumption. It makes me sick to my stomach when I hear parents say they make Macaroni and Cheese for their children’s dinner because it’s “easy.” You’re right, it is easy to damage your child's brain, have inflammation run rampant in their body, and give them a leaky gut. Grains are particularly more dangerous for children because their bodies are still developing. If they get a bad signal from the food they eat that gets replicated and programmed over and over, this is how childhood obesity thrives, and diabetes becomes the new killer of people under the age of 10.

Long story short, STOP FEEDING GRAINS TO YOUR KIDS! I don't care how healthy that box of cereal promotes itself to be, the wording and advertisements are designed to sell you their product. If you don't care to stop feeding your children bread, cereal, or pasta then don't be surprised when they are staying home sick instead of going to school. Don't be surprised by their lack of motivation to learn or their weight gain. Easy is a trickster. Your child needs traditionally cooked food like eggs, a grass fed hamburger, grass fed butter-drenched broccoli or mashed cauliflower. They need avocado, bacon, and steak tossed into an arugula salad, not pizza parties every weekend, sandwiched between pasta filled weeknights because of the ease it provides feeding your child. Kill the soda and fruit juice and give them a green smoothie or a Kombucha (Fermented tea), which provides them with living nutrients rather than phosphoric acid and caramel coloring. If you want a healthy productive child feed them well!

Client Story Maya's Daughter

I apologize for that little rant, but you have not seen some of the heartbreaking cases I have dealt with over my time. While in a gym in Hawai'i a lady by the name of Maya overheard me talking to another member about nutrition. Intrigued she asked me about my schooling and seemingly passing her test of approval she asked me if I could help her with her daughter. I said of course and she went on to explain to me that she is a single mom working nearly 12 hours a day as a nurse so she leaves her 8-year-old daughter with her parents nearly all day every work day. Her parents, lacking the desire to control their grandchild's nutrition have effectively grown her 8-year-old daughter to 180lbs.! She gets cereal and pancakes for breakfast, cookies and noodles for lunch, and then rice, macaroni salad, and a small amount of chicken for dinner followed by all the ice cream she can eat. Maya was lost. She didn't know what to do or how to talk to her parents about the troubling weight gain her child was experiencing. I explained to her that not only were her parents feeding her daughter copious amounts of sugar, but the lectins in the grains being eaten at every meal is also opening up her body to infection, autoimmune disease, and potentially diabetes in the near future. My advice to her was two fold:

1. Throw out everything in a box or a bag in her parent's home.

2. I gave her one of my allowable food lists and told her to have them hang it on the fridge and her daughter is to only eat those specific foods for breakfast, lunch, and dinner.

Being as passionate as I am about the subject, I also instructed her to look her parents dead in the eye and sternly request that they stop killing her child! Putting her newfound plan into action Maya's daughter was down an amazing 30lbs. after 6 weeks. She was happier, more energetic and outgoing, and playing more with the other kids in her school. Maya was grateful of the quick reversal her daughter was experiencing and had also created a better understanding of nutrition for her parents. She no longer worries about leaving her daughter when going to work!

Today, more than 70% of American adults are overweight, and of those 70% almost 38% are obese (16). This is all thanks to the heart healthy grain veil that has been pulled over our eyes by the one-two punch of Dr. Ancel Keys, and Senator George McGovern. Are these two men evil? Did they hatch a plan to try and destroy the very country they were born in? Absolutely not. They were simply men with a job to do trying to make a difference with what they believed was right at the time. As you can see with the second edition of this book coming a little over one year after it was first released, our understanding of nutrition changes very rapidly. My hope is that the new research travels fast. I would love to wake up one day and hear people talking about how eliminating grains in their nutrition has changed their life. I want to hear stories on NBC, CNN, and the like. I want to read about it in magazines. I'd love to hear mothers talking about how they removed grains from their child's nutrition and experienced phenomenal results. I want to hear someone acknowledge her as if to say, “Duh, we all know grains contain lectins and are not good to consume.”

Unfortunately we are just not there yet, and this book is all I can do to present the correct information to those searching for it. If you have tried many other diets in the past and nothing has seemed to work, you may want to try eliminating all lectin containing food from your nutritional arsenal. These silent killers may have been what were holding you back!

Lectin Containing Foods:

- Whole grain pasta
- Brown Rice
- Potatoes
- Milk
- Whole grain breads
- Tortillas
- Cookies
- Crackers
- Cereal
- Peas
- Sugar snap peas
- Legumes
- Green beans
- Chickpeas
- Soy
- Tofu
- Edamame
- Sprouts

- Lentils
- Quinoa
- Pumpkin seeds
- Sunflower seeds
- Chia seeds
- Peanuts
- Cashews
- Cucumbers
- Zucchini
- Squashes
- Melons
- Eggplant
- Tomatoes
- Bell peppers
- Chili peppers
- Gogi berries
- Grain fed animal meat
- Oats
- Corn/Corn products

Sorry I'm not sorry about the long list, but your health matters to me. Before we get back to regular ol' chapter 2, as a parting gift I'd like to share with you the diseases we are finding out lectins may be causing in the human body. This includes but is not limited to:

- Obesity
- Cancer
- Type 2 diabetes
- Coronary heart disease
- Celiac disease

- Influenza (by destroying the mucosal lining in the small intestine)
- Irritable bowel syndrome
- Lupus
- Multiple sclerosis
- Rheumatoid arthritis
- Lymphomas
- Multiple myelomas
- Crohn's disease
- Ulcerative colitis
- Fibromyalgia
- Pretty much every autoimmune disease

Even though this list is not as daunting as the list of diseases milk provides, it still is a pretty nasty list. I don't know anyone that would be willing to tolerate a lymphoma just to have his or her daily bowl of whole grains. To me, the solution is simple, it's not what you eat that makes you sick, it what you choose not to eat that keeps you healthy. Do not let lectins destroy your health and ultimately your happiness!

Fruits (Back to Chapter 2)

Surely there are worse things you can put in your body than fruit, right? Yes and no. Remember how I mentioned earlier that fruit does not send a signal to our brain telling us we are full? Well the full story is even worse. Fruits have long told animals and humans alike that their color is associated with ripeness. Red, yellow, and orange colors have said, "Eat me, I'm ready for you to take my seeds and deposit them somewhere else so my babies can grow." When a fruit is ripe, it also reduces the amount of lectins it has in its skin and seeds. The problem these days is that fruits are picked slightly unripe and then they are sprayed with ethylene oxide when they arrive at their destination to change the color of the skin only, making them appear ripe and ready to buy. The consumer unknowingly buys the ripe fruit (which is unripe inside) takes it home and eats it consuming higher than normal lectins. This becomes a huge detriment to your health!

The people who sing fruits praises want to say that the fiber that the fruit contains slow the digestion of fructose. This may be true, but the problem that we see is two fold. One, the sugar in the fruit, regardless of how slow it digests, will still create an insulin response that we don't want in the body. Two, just because something has fiber accompanying the sugar does not make it healthy to eat. Is a donut ok for me to eat as long as I chase it down with a glass of Metamucil? Heck no! The sad fact is that the general public is sold that fruit is very nutritious and should be eaten every day. Is it the reason why people are fat, or get fat? No. Is it the reason why people have a difficult time losing fat/weight? YES! Check out the chart below. Everyone knows fruit juice is better for you than soda, right? Guess again! Look at the sugar concentration of your sons grape juice you're serving him:

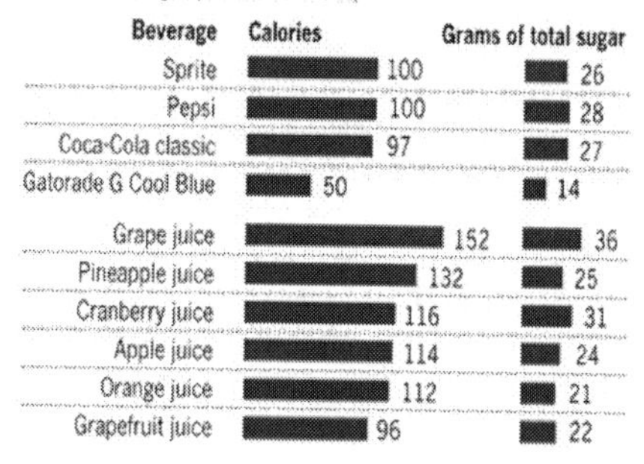

Fruit juice vs. soft drinks

Juice enjoys the reputation of a health food, but critics say its calorie and sugar content are on a par with soda and other more vilified beverages.

Calorie and sugar counts of selected beverages

(Per 8-ounce serving; all juices are unsweetened)

Beverage	Calories	Grams of total sugar
Sprite	100	26
Pepsi	100	28
Coca-Cola classic	97	27
Gatorade G Cool Blue	50	14
Grape juice	152	36
Pineapple juice	132	25
Cranberry juice	116	31
Apple juice	114	24
Orange juice	112	21
Grapefruit juice	96	22

Sources: U.S. Department of Agriculture Nutrient Data Laboratory; company information
Graphics reporting by KAREN KAPLAN

Los Angeles Times

Now look at the relative sweetness of fructose compared to other sugars:

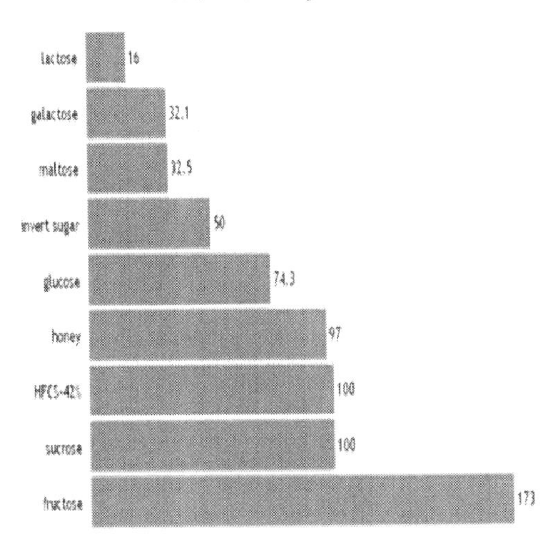

Fruits and fruit juices are driven by the carbohydrate industry as a great way to start off your day. But the problem is that this is another health PERCEPTION. Having any type of sugar, especially fructose for breakfast, signals our pancreas to start producing insulin to grab all of that sugar in the blood and most likely store it. As you'll read, this spells big trouble for us!

Insulin: It's What's For Breakfast

Picture yourself as a healthy man or woman, about 160lbs and 30% body fat. You go on a diet and soon find yourself down to 28% body fat, then 22% body fat, and then 18%. This usually will happen over the course of 4-6 months. Great right? But then you measure your body fat and it's 23%. You had a feeling it went up because you could see it in the mirror. Then back up to 25% a month later. You're doing everything the same in the gym, eating according to the guidelines. What's happening? Insulin, that's what!

Usually when we eat processed foods, (by processed I'm talking about cereal, cookies, pasta; foods that do not normally occur in nature, but instead are created on a whiteboard in some company's laboratory); our body regards them as very toxic and stores most of it as fat. We go on a diet and since we are not eating anymore-processed foods, we lose the toxins and fat that our body stored previously. Now, if you're familiar with diet and exercise, you know eating carbohydrates causes an increase in insulin in the body. When we wake up, our body releases an adrenal hormone called cortisol. Normally, in the human body, only one, cortisol, or insulin is released, never both at the same time. Eating carbohydrates for breakfast causes the pancreas to release insulin, and insulin, in the presence of cortisol signals the brain to make NEW fat cells! So the fruit smoothie you made for breakfast this morning just told your body to make new fat cells. The scary fact is that a fat cell has only one job and that is to get full! So it starts sending out signals to the brain for more sugar, more carbs, until it is nice and full and happy, hence the fat/weight that we regain.

What Else Does Insulin Do?

Insulin is a hormone that comes from your pancreas. It has many different jobs in the human body. The more we test insulin, the more we find out, as it is responsible for many, many things in the human body. Insulin can and will:

- Absorb sugar in the blood and partition it to the muscle or fat cell.
- Help replicate DNA and synthesize protein when present.
- Help uptake amino acids, utilize potassium and increase enzymatic activity.
- Increase blood flow.
- Decrease protein breakdown.
- Lowers the rate of fat burning and gluconeogenesis (the generation of sugar from non carbohydrate sources).
- Bind to the kidneys and signal them to excrete calcium in the urine (5).

The previous list is just what insulin likes to do in its spare time, sort of like hormone hobbies. The main role of insulin, what it is really there for, is to keep the body in an anabolic (muscle building) state as it triggers the growth of everything.

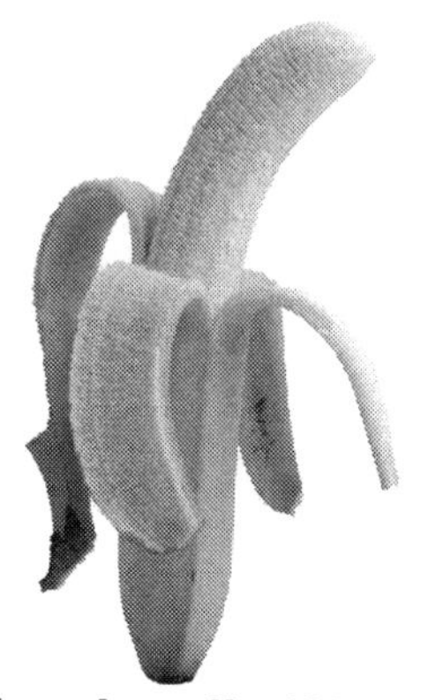

How Insulin Works

For the scope of this guide, we will simplify the terms of how insulin works for a universal understanding. To do this, we will use a........... Banana! Every person in the world that wakes up in the morning wakes up burning fat for fuel. What we eat after that dictates whether or not our body continues to burn fat or whether or not that process gets disrupted by presence of carbohydrates. See the following example pertaining to two people:

Person #1 – Wakes up at 7:30am for work and has a cup of coffee with two over easy eggs and 3 pieces of bacon. This person continues to burn fat until their next meal since no carbohydrates were introduced.

Person #2 – Wakes up at 7:30am for work and has a banana and a cup of coffee. Once the fructose from the sugar in the banana reaches the blood stream, the pancreas releases insulin to go scoop it up. As soon as insulin is released the body stops burning fat for fuel, and forces the consumed sugar to be used as fuel. Because person #2 is commuting to work and not doing any physical activity, insulin takes the sugar directly to fat cells for storage to be used at a later date. The fat burning process has been disrupted and the brain now realizes it needs more "quick fuel." Before you know it, person #2 is reaching for more food.

As you can see, person #2 is on the fast track to fluffiness. Person #2 will not only consume more sugar throughout the day in all of its forms, but probably more calories as well. Consuming mostly fat, protein, and fibrous or low glycemic vegetables during the day, then consuming your lean meats and higher glycemic vegetables in the evening avoids all this.

So should fruits be avoided all together? No. There are certain fruits we find have resistant starches in them that feed out good gut bacteria. A list of them will be in the nutritional guides section. We are led to believe that we NEED fruit in order to survive, that it is ESSENTIAL to our health. The truth is that it is not. I have about one, maybe two pieces of fruit a MONTH and I have no health complications at all. If I do eat fruit it will be at night when my body can't store the sugar as fat, or I'll eat it 30 minutes before a workout so the sugar gets used as fuel. This is how we get the benefit of fruit, without the negative insulin raising effects.

Bottom line is that fruit is just as bad as candy. Don't believe me because I'm not a doctor? Well here is a quote from one:

"Modern Fruit is as bad as candy."

~ Dr. Stephen Gundry, *The Plant Paradox.*

How can fruit be bad? Well as we discussed earlier, fructose does not send a signal to your brain telling you to stop eating. From an evolutionary standpoint this allowed us to eat an unlimited amount of sugar to fatten up for the coming winter so we wouldn't starve to death. Due to the fact that there are very few people starving to death in the U.S. these days fruit has become more of an enemy than a friend. Unbeknownst to all you fruit loving shoppers out there fructose is quickly become the primary reason for most kidney failures doctors are seeing. Fructose is so toxic that 60 percent of what is digested is shoveled directly to the liver where it is converted into triglycerides (which are a marker for heart disease) and uric acid, which raises blood pressure, causes gout, and directly damages your kidneys' ability to filtrate your blood (20). Your liver is the garbage dump of your body, filtering out all toxins to keep you health and alive. What is that saying if 60% of a nutrient in the food you just ate went straight into the garbage?

Don't get me wrong; I am not a fruit hater. What I do hate is the perception commercials and advertisements promoting fruit portray. It's a smiling woman, or active, healthy looking kids crushing a massive glass of juice in the morning.

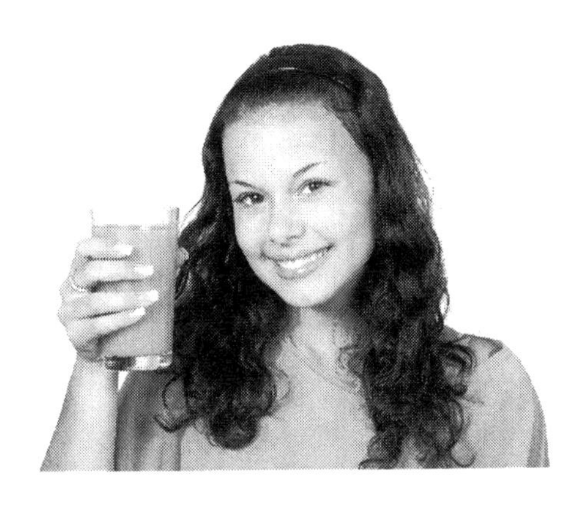

Here's to a cracked out liver y'all!

If the research and information I'm stating here is still not enough to deter you from your sweet glass of O.J., then here's my final challenge – buy the oranges, and juice them yourself! This will at least ensure its just lovely oranges in your glass and no preservatives or deteriorated forms of calcium and vitamin D.

Now that I have you all feathered from the facts, I'm going to stay true to my anti-reductionist nature and recommend some fruits I feel are better than others if you ever get a craving for a sweet natural treat:

Apples – Strengthen our teeth, and aid in digestion.

Avocados – helps balance our good and bad cholesterol.

Bananas – Has anti-fungal, and antibiotic properties. Make sure to only eat them when they are green so you are introducing resistant starches to your good gut bacteria.

Figs & Dates – Contain fructooligosaccharides (FOS), which is a form of indigestible sugar that your good gut bacteria thrive on. Interesting fact, figs are flowers not fruit which gives them a huge thumbs up!

Green Mangoes – Full of resistant starches, which provide extreme satiety and feed only your good gut bacteria.

Green Papaya - Full of resistant starches, which provide extreme satiety and feed only your good gut bacteria.

Green Plantains - Full of resistant starches, which provide extreme satiety and feed only your good gut bacteria.

Grapes – Has antiviral properties.

Oranges – Stimulate digestion, and alleviates constipation.

Tangerines – Contain synephrine, a natural decongestant that can help clear the lungs.

So much of how we use food (especially fruit) comes down to the timing of consuming it. Not only do certain foods create unfavorable reactions in our body, but also the reaction may be even more pronounced if it is consumed at the wrong point in the day. Through the use of carb loading, which you will learn about shortly, it seems that we can have our cake and eat it, so long as it's at a certain point in the day and it will not affect our hormonal system the way it normally does. Hormones rise and fall throughout the day and are also influenced by food. With the help of science you will soon find out what makes my nutrition program so unique!

Milk

Wondering why milk is in the carbohydrate section? Because it is all SUGAR! Look at the nutrition labels on all of your favorite milk drinks:

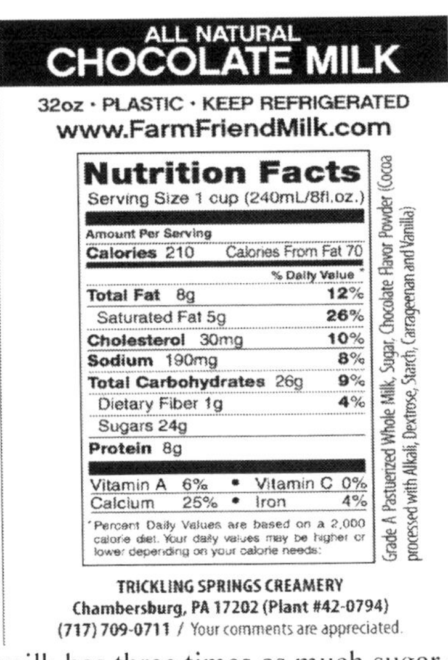

Chocolate milk has three times as much sugar as it does fat.

Strawberry Milk

Nutrition Facts
Serving Size 1 Cup (240mL)

Amount Per Serving	
Calories 190	Calories from Fat 70
	% Daily Value*
Total Fat 8g	**12%**
Saturated Fat 5g	**25%**
Trans Fat 0g	**0%**
Cholesterol 30mg	**10%**
Sodium 125mg	**5%**
Total Carbohydrate 22g	**7%**
Dietary Fiber 0g	
Sugars 22g	
Protein 7g	

Vitamin A 10% • Vitamin C 6%
Calcium 50% • Iron 0% • Vitamin E 25%
Percent Daily Values are based on a 2000 calorie diet.

Strawberry milk again has three times as much sugar as it does fat or protein.

Whole Milk

Serving Size 8 fl oz (240mL)
Servings Per Container 2

Amount Per Serving	
Calories 150	Calories from Fat 70
	% Daily Value*
Total Fat 8g	12%
Saturated Fat 5g	25%
Cholesterol 35mg	12%
Sodium 125mg	5%
Total Carbohydrate 12g	4%
Dietary Fiber 0g	0%
Sugars 11g	
Protein 8g	

Whole milk is much more balanced. Still a lot of sugar, but it has higher amounts of fat, especially saturated fat that would keep you fuller for longer.

2% REDUCED-FAT MILK Nutrition Facts	
Serving Size 1 cup (240 ml) Servings Per Container 8	
Amount Per Serving	
Calories 120	Calories from Fat 45
	% Daily Value
Total Fat 5g	8%
Saturated Fat 3 g	15%
Cholesterol 50 mg	17%
Sodium 125mg	5%
Total Carbohydrate 12 g	4%
Dietary Fiber0g	0%
Sugars 11g	
Protein 8g	

2% milk, which is a definite favorite, is coming in at twice as much sugar as fat, and 1.5 times as much sugar as protein.

SKIM MILK

Nutrition Facts

Serving Size 1 cup (240mL)
Servings Per Container 16

Amount Per Serving

Calories 80	Calories from Fat 0
	% Daily Value*
Total Fat 0g	0%
Saturated Fat 0g	0%
Trans Fat 0g	
Cholesterol 0mg	0%
Sodium 120mg	5%
Total Carbohydrate 11g	4%
Dietary Fiber 0g	0%
Sugars 11g	
Protein 8g	

Vitamin A 0% • Vitamin C 6%
Calcium 30% • Iron 0%
Vitamin D 25% •

* Percent Daily Values are based on a 2,000 calorie diet. Your daily values may be higher or lower depending on your calorie needs:

	Calories:	2,000	2,500
Total Fat	Less than	65g	80g
Sat Fat	Less than	20g	25g
Cholesterol	Less than	300mg	300mg
Sodium	Less than	2,400mg	2,400mg
Total Carbohydrate		300g	375g
Dietary Fiber		25g	30g

Calories per gram:
Fat 9 • Carbohydrate 4 • Protein 4

Skim milk has 11 times more sugar than fat, and 1.5 times as much sugar as protein.

Milk is an $11 Billion dollar a year industry, and cheese is $16 billion dollars in just the U.S. alone. In 2003, Dairy management Inc. put together what they call a unified marketing plan to keep Americans consuming dairy products regardless of the negative effects its has on our health. In 2003, their budget was $165 million, so they definitely mean business. All of this money was directed at one thing, to "protect and enhance consumer confidence in dairy products and the dairy industry. A large part of this program aims to reach children between the ages of 6-12 years old, and their mothers, in hopes that they will be dairy consumers for life. I tell people that most of our food is designed by manufacturers to keep us addicted, but what the dairy industry does is just plain wrong. Please keep reading.

What many people don't know is how contaminated the milk sources are. They are commonly tainted with disease-causing bacteria such as salmonella, staphylococci, listeria, deadly E. coli O1573 and Mycobacterium paratuberculosis (possibly one of the agents causing Crohn's disease; a form of life-threatening chronic colitis), as well as virus's known to cause lymphoma and leukemia-like diseases, and immune deficiency in cattle (4). The milk we consume also has acceptable levels of pus in it regulated by the FDA. When we consume milk, our body must make pus to combat the pus. This produces inflammation and distracts the immune system from protecting the body from disease so we have a tendency to get sick more often. Even with pasteurization, there are fragments of viruses that get into the milk we consume that may be even more dangerous to our health (4).

There is also a mutated protein in milk called A-1 beta casein. This mutated protein can sneak through the intestinal wall when it is not yet fully developed (such as in children aged 6-12). The immune system will then make antibodies to combat the protein, but the problem is that this protein also attacks the cells of the pancreas. If the child continues to consume too much diary, diabetes ensues. This is the major issue going on lately, but there are many, many other diseases that are linked to dairy consumption. Here's a list I got from Dr. McDougall's newsletter, if you don't understand something, just throw it in Google as explanation of every one of these diseases is beyond the scope of this book.

Upper Gastrointestinal:

- Canker sores (aphthous stomatitis)
- Irritation of tongue, lips and mouth
- Tonsil enlargement
- Vomiting
- Gastro esophageal reflux (GERD)
- Sandifer's syndrome
- Peptic ulcer disease
- Colic
- Stomach cramps
- Abdominal distention
- Intestinal obstruction
- Type-1 diabetes

Lower Gastrointestinal:

- Bloody stools
- Colitis
- Malabsorption of food
- Diarrhea
- Painful defecation
- Fecal soiling
- Infantile colic
- Chronic constipation
- Infantile food protein-induced enterocolitis syndrome Crohn's disease
- Ulcerative colitis.

Respiratory:

- Nasal stuffiness Runny nose
- Otitis media (inner ear trouble)
- Sinusitis
- Wheezing
- Asthma
- Pulmonary infiltrates

Bone and joint:

- Rheumatoid arthritis
- Juvenile rheumatoid arthritis
- Lupus

- Beheta's disease

Skin:

- Rashes
- Atopic dermatitis
- Eczema
- Seborrhea
- Hives
- Acne

Nervous System (Behavioral):

- Multiple sclerosis
- Parkinson's disease
- Autism
- Schizophrenia
- Irritability
- Restlessness
- Hyperactivity
- Headache
- Allergic-tension fatigue syndrome
- Muscle pain
- Depression
- Enuresis (bed-wetting).

Blood:

- Abnormal blood clotting
- Iron deficiency anemia
- Low serum proteins

- Thrombocytopenia
- Eosinophilia

Other:

- Nephrotic syndrome
- Glomerulonephritis
- Anaphylactic shock and death
- Sudden infant death syndrome
- Injury to the arteries causing arteritis, and eventually, atherosclerosis.

This is just a SMALL list! For a more complete list go to www.notmilk.com and prepare to be horrified. I'd like to share another personal story about my experience with milk. It was June of 2013 and life could not have been better. I woke up one day with a wicked stomachache, but after my morning coffee and a little bit of exercise, everything went back to normal. Then it happened the next day, and the next day, and then every day was like that! Worried, as this is not the norm for me I tried to trouble shoot. I stopped drinking alcohol, I stopped eating sugar, and I started eating only organic foods. Nothing seemed to work.

Soon thereafter, I started to get pain in my knuckles. Being a coach, athlete, and body worker, my hands mean everything to me! I started to search the Internet relentlessly for the answer and everything kept pointing to milk! The fact was that I did not consume very much milk at all, but what I did consume was a lion's share of heavy cream in my coffee every morning!

I would pour close to two inches of heavy cream in my coffee because the casein in cream is extremely slow to digest so it would stop me from being hungry all morning while I was coaching. As I kept reading and researching, one very interesting article mentioned that when detoxifying from milk, you will lose over a pound of mucus from your body. Remember earlier we talked about there being pus in the milk we consume and how our body must make mucus to combat it? Well they weren't lying because when I quit milk cold turkey, I was coughing up major amounts of phlegm for over 4 weeks! In the meantime, my stomachaches went away, and my knuckles also stopped hurting soon thereafter.

A friend of mine saw all the effects of the detox and decided to jump on the no milk kick with me. The crazy thing was that she saw an even more amazing change! She has had sneezing fits her entire life. When she was young she told me that her and her Dad would consume almost an entire gallon of milk a day! She grew up sickly, having very many visits to the doctor for a multitude of different things. As she also detoxed off of milk, her sneezing fits decreased by 10 times the usual. We tested this many times where she would be fine all day, no sneezing, then we would give her a small piece of chocolate. Not even 3 minutes later she was sneezing her head off, and her nose would get stuffed. As of this writing, it's been two years since quitting milk and she has been basically symptom free. She just went and got an allergy test from her doctor, and it showed a sensitivity to milk, not an allergy so her body is reversing the damage done which is exciting.

Now, I know many of you may be screaming, "But I need to get my calcium!" The fact is that the body requires many vitamins and nutrients to make new bone, specifically vitamin D and vitamin K2. I recommend taking between 5-15,000I.U. of vitamin D a day in the supplement section, and you can get plenty of vitamin K in organ meats, egg yolks, organic ground beef, broccoli, spinach, and other green, leafy vegetables. It appears that when vitamin D and K are present with protein, calcium is pulled from the blood to simulate bone formation (5).

Vitamin D does many amazing things, but it looks like it also tells the kidneys to reabsorb calcium as well. With all of this calcium being reabsorbed, this makes the 30% of your daily value you receive from a glass of milk less significant. You may want to reconsider calcium supplementation as well as studies are showing it is not absorbed and used by the body very well, and in fact when portions of a blocked coronary artery were removed from a heart attack patient, most of the contents was calcium, not cholesterol (5). For these reasons alone, we should not be concerned with missing the calcium milk provides when we get plenty of it elsewhere and our body even recycles it. I bet the dairy industry was hoping no one would find that out. Think about that next time you drive past a billboard with a smiling child donning a milk mustache!

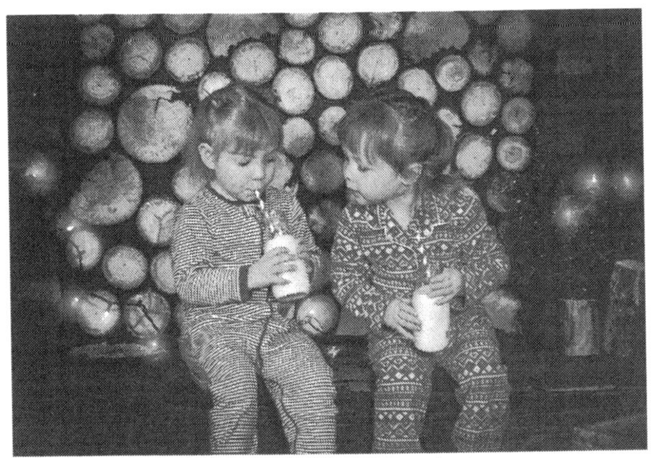
Hey, yours has more pus in it than mine!

Giving up dairy products is not easy because milk is in EVERYTHING! Bottom line is being smart. Check the label on all carbohydrate products regardless of what it is, you'll be surprised what they sneak milk into nowadays!

Teenage Mutant Ninja.....Cows?

I mentioned this earlier, but would like to discuss in a little bit greater depth for you now. As much as I tried to find a solid number, the debate is still ongoing as to when a spontaneous mutation occurred in cows turning a protein they have called casein into a deadly lectin-like structure known as beta-casomorphin. Some researchers have said 10,000 years, and others say 2,000 years. In all reality, the time does not matter, what matters is this fun little guy likes to attach itself to the cells that make insulin in your pancreas and is thought of by some forward thinkers in the health field as the true cause of type 1 diabetes. Just when you thought the case against milk couldn't get any dimmer, I drop that one on you. But there is hope and that's the only reason I'm telling you this story.

The cows with the mutation are primarily black and white Holstein cows scientifically categorized as A-1 cows. Their brown and white cousins have somehow survived this mutation (Which scientists have dubbed the A-2 cow) and some stores have started carrying this type of milk. Manufactured by the A-2 milk company based out of New Zealand, this may be a better alternative to your regular organic cows milk if you just can't let it go. I still advise against drinking copious amounts of even A-2 milk especially consuming it on a daily basis because of the possibility of high pus content, but this definitely is an option if the mood strikes you for a nice white mustache.

There's a book called *The Slight Edge* written by Jeff Olson in which he describes how making a bunch of good small decisions, then one bad decision will barely affect you at all. However, the inverse is not true. Making a ton of bad decision and then one good decision does not make you a hero. I want you to think about this in regards to your food choices as well. As you'll find out later, "eating clean" does not have to be a round the clock thing. There will be times where the white glove of food snobbiness can come off and you can indulge because this one bad food choice will barely affect your internal environment. We just have to do the work of getting to that point first, and this is where the beauty of my program shines because you literally trick your brain into thinking it is not on a diet. When we have control over the food we eat, having a glass of A-2 milk, or a piece from a lectin bomb birthday cake will barely affect us because we have that slight edge!

Fiber

As stated previously, fiber intake during evolutionary times was very high. Today it is very low. How much is needed lies somewhere in between that and depends on the individual. With all of the processed foods nowadays that are void of fiber, one of the greatest shifts an overweight individual can make is eating more fibrous vegetables, instead of the refined carbohydrates in a box or a bag. Here is the best list of fiber benefits I could find to date (from http://www.bodyrecomposition.com):

- Promotes fullness/satiety
- Slows gastric emptying
- Decreases nutrient absorption
- Improves sugar control
- Decreases blood cholesterol
- Decreases mineral absorption
- Positive effects on insulin sensitivity
- A number of positive effects relevant to colon cancer
- Helps with poopin'

A pretty interesting effect primarily seen with soluble fibers is it impairs nutrient absorption for carbohydrates, fats and dietary protein. When fiber is digested there is a gel-like mass that is formed that digestive enzymes can't get access to, and as a result the other nutrients end up getting carried out of the body. This means that high-fiber diets will result in less total caloric absorption, but not by much. Fiber may reduce total fat absorption by about 3%, protein by 5%, and there is no solid number found for carbohydrates at the moment, it's probably just as small. Just so you get a clear idea of what we are talking about, an increase in dietary fiber in your diet from 18 to 36 grams per day might reduce total caloric absorption by 100 calories per day. Small, but in some cases it may be worth it.

Now, depending on how you want to look at this, it can be seen as either a good or bad thing. For individuals trying to lose weight, higher fiber diets will not only have positive effects on fullness, but will result in less total calories being absorbed from the diet. If weight gain is your goal, high fiber intake may not be the best course of action, but won't be as detrimental as some others may say. Lastly, many experts have been known to say that fiber is zero calories or may actually have a negative calorie value and this simply is not true. While there is still some debate in the area, researchers are assigning a value of 1.5-2.0 calories/gram to most fibers.

Fermented Foods

Amazingly, as far back as recorded history goes, human beings have been eating fermented foods. Scientists in the mid to late 1800's were studying the efficacy of fermented foods and started to credit them with being immune system boosters and increasing life expectancy. Here are some great historical facts about fermented foods before we get to the nitty gritty of why you want to eat them:

- 5400 BCE – Winemaking in Iran
- 5000 BCE – Milk fermentation in Babylon
- 4000 BCE – Fermented cabbage in China
- 3000 BCE – Leaven bread in Egypt
- 2000 BCE – Pulque, the oldest alcoholic beverage on the North American continent, which originated in Mexico! (11)
- 76 CE – Roman Historian Plinio discovers fermented milk helps with gastro intestinal problems

Those are just some of the historical facts of fermented foods, I'm sure if we really researched there are thousands of others.

What are Fermented Foods?

Fermented foods are created when we introduce natural bacteria or yeast to food, and it then feeds on the sugar in the food fermenting it. There are several different kinds of fermented foods we can enjoy.

- Cultured Veggies – legumes are cooked and hulled to make tempeh.

- Meat flavored pastes – soybeans are mashed and left to ferment to make pastes and sauces. Examples are soy sauce, miso, shoyu, Vietnamese mam, and Malaysian belachan.

- Alcohol Fermentations – Wine, rum, whiskey, vodka, beer.

- Vinegar Fermentations – Our beloved apple cider vinegar, coconut water vinegar, and wine vinegars.

- Alkaline Fermented Foods – Japanese Natto made from cooked soybeans.

- Leavened Breads – These are made from fermented grains and include rye and sourdough bread. (These are the only two types of bread I will ever eat)

- Lactic Acid Fermentation – Bacteria convert's sugars present in the food to cellular energy and lactic acid, thus preserving it naturally. These include sauerkraut, pickles, olives, kimchi, kefir, yogurt, cheeses and tofu.

Why Do We Want to Eat Fermented Foods?

Currently, in the United States alone, there are over 190 million doses of antibiotics administered PER DAY, and more than 133 million courses of antibiotics are prescribed by doctors to non-hospitalized patients per year (11)! Not only is that alarming, because most of these illnesses are caused by a poor diet and should be reversed by a correct diet, but in addition to killing off bad bacteria, antibiotics kill off a lot of good bacteria too. Consider this, there are 10 trillion cells in the human body, yet there are 100 trillion bacteria cells living IN our body! This is why it is bad for us to take antibiotics, because the balance of good to bad bacteria is essential for our health. Your good gut bacteria love to feed on fermented foods, resistant starches, and cruciferous veggies while your bad gut bacteria thrive on sugar and its derivatives. Which ever are thriving at the moment – good or bad is who will send the strongest signal to you for what it wants to eat. Oh I'm sorry, you thought you were choosing what you want to eat? Not so!

Feeding your good gut bacteria means that you will actually crave the foods that are good for you, this is why it is so important to keep that *Slight Edge* in your life when it come to your nutrition. The more correct decisions we make, the easier it is to keep making good decisions on what we eat! Cravings disappear, fat dissolves as we sleep, and a leaner, happier person starts to evolve, and fermented foods are a huge contributor to this.

Eating fermented foods essentially replaces the need for antibiotics as well. They provide enzymes, which help digest our food easier and increase our life span, as well as increase the amount of usable vitamins in our food by 5 – 10 times the normal amount! Also, any babies that are born by C-section miss picking up the bacteria in the mother's birth canal and can have a weak immune system later in life. Fermented foods strengthen our immune system by neutralizing endo-toxins, which are what the bad bacteria defend themselves with, and they, increase the amount of cytokines our body produces, which is our way of defending bad bacteria. Eighty percent of our immune system resides in our small intestine. Why? Because that is the first area INSIDE the body! Most people think it is the stomach, but the stomach is still the outside of the body considering if I eat something that doesn't agree with me I can throw it up. Once something foreign enters the small intestine it can diffuse through the intestinal wall and into the blood then BAM, we're sick. So it is very important that our immune system is healthy and on high alert for new viruses, rather than battling bad bacteria flourishing and running amuck because our nutrition is terrible.

Fermented foods are also amazing for the prevention of certain diseases. As I mentioned earlier, Cancer is now being looked at and treated as a metabolic disease. This means that it starts with a poor diet. Fermented foods neutralize carcinogenic nitrites in our processed foods, especially meats (more on this in the protein section). They also extract calcium from dairy products so the body can better utilize it, and it helps us digest fiber. Here is a short list of other diseases fermented foods can help reverse or cure:

- Leaky gut syndrome
- Heartburn
- Ulcers
- Irritable bowel syndrome
- Crohn's disease (ulcers in the GI tract)
- Arthritis
- Psoriasis
- Asthma
- Autism

- Multiple Sclerosis

I don't know about you, but once again that is a list of diseases I hope I never experience. The bottom line is that fermented foods are just too important not to eat. I eat some type of fermented food at least once a day (my favs are kimchi, sauerkraut, and apple cider vinegar). I realize some of them are made from soy and milk, which I tell you not to eat in this book, but by fermenting, we can make a poor nutrient a good one. Fermented soy products are the only type of soy I would put in my body. Drinking soymilk by the gallon or eating fresh soybeans every day are a no-no because it wreaks havoc on the hormonal system of both men and women alike. It should be a crime to sell such things but every time I go into the store there they are sitting on the shelf.

To wrap up, I would start off eating fermented food with at least one meal per day. Then move to two and so on. I've noticed a big improvement in how I feel when I have my morning sausage with sauerkraut than without it, or I'll have a hamburger patty with kimchi. Digestion is better and I feel more energetic. All you have to do is introduce them slowly, and they do grow on you. You're talking to a guy who used to turn his nose up at sauerkraut and now has a constant supply of it in his fridge!

Kombucha: A great alternative to soda!

I stumbled upon this little gem back in 2011 when I was at the supermarket buying my lunch and craving something bubbly. I looked feverishly through the massive amount of canned and bottled beverages looking for a diamond in the ruff. It seemed as if everything either had too much sugar, or not enough carbonation. Just when I was ready to give up, I landed my eyes on Gt's Kombucha. Bubbly? Check! Sugar low? Check! How can this be? I bought it, and fell in love on the first sip.

Just recently when polled, 63% of Americans said they are making the switch and cutting soda out of their diet. I realize the manufacturers who created soda made it to be addictive, hence the great taste and us wanting to go back for more, but seriously, who ever thought caramel coloring, phosphoric acid, and carbonated water would be the epitome of thirst quenching? The marketing ploys for soda are genius. Geniusly evil! When the whole high fructose corn syrup rebellion started Coca-Cola put their soda back in their original glass bottle and called it Coca-Cola Life because of their switch back to real sugar! Life!!!! I assure you no life can survive in that bottle, nor will it be giving life to anyone who drinks it.

Mexico is the last country that has been suffering at the perils of soda and fruit juice. The massive increase in type 2 diabetes diagnoses of their children is believed by scientists to be caused by you guessed it – soda consumption. Scientists actually believe the problem is two fold because some of the children (children now!) are showing sign of having a fatty liver – which is the early onset of cirrhosis, a disease seen frequently in alcoholics! Scientists believe it is the high consumption of both soda, and fruit in combination that is waging war on these young n's insides.

When I advise mothers to cut all cows milk, soda, and fruit juice from their child's diet, I often get shrieks of horror, and looks of disgust from them. "What am I supposed to give him/her to drink then?" is their reply. I suggest water or Kombucha throughout the day, and coffee in the morning bulletproof style, or with some heavy cream. Their head now looks ready to implode from incomprehension. "Coffee! You would give a child coffee?" You mean would I give a child a naturally caffeinated beverage that comes from the Earth bursting with polyphenols that have numerous health benefits. Yes. Yes I would. Start him or her with decaf, and then slowly introduce regular coffee. Serve it iced, or hot. Everyone has been to Starbucks - use your imagination, the multitude of choices is endless! You can use unsweetened almond, or coconut milk to make a late`. Blend butter in there with coconut oil Bulletproof style! Find something your child likes and get them in the habit of craving it when looking for a beverage. You'll thank me, I promise!

Ok, sorry about that sidebar, back to Kombucha. Kombucha is fermented tea. Through the fermentation process the scoby feeds on the sugar in the tea and creates good bacteria, and carbonation, which creates a lovely soda-like concoction. When Kombucha first hit the shelves in stores around 2011, they were sold with names like gingerade, or green machine (Now there are many, many more flavors) and contained around 2-4 grams of sugar per serving (4-8 grams total) compared to soda and its average of 46 grams of sugar per can or bottle. Everyone I have convinced to make the switch has fallen in love with Kombucha and feels the difference this healthy probiotic creates for their insides. If you scour the Internet however, you will find some people that it just does not agree with. Common irritations can be bloating and excessive gas. If this is you, an alternative is to put a dash of Bragg's apple cider vinegar inside a cup of filtered water, which creates the same type of gut enhancing benefits.

A word of caution about store bought Kombucha. Due to its rise in popularity manufacturers are now starting to create several more flavors whilst sneaking more sugar in per serving. I've seen some brands climbing as high as 12-16 grams of sugar per serving (Times 2 servings per bottle which is 24-36 grams total and getting close to our beloved soda count!). As Kombucha gains more of a following, manufacturers will start to compete for your taste buds – hence the added sugar. A great way to combat this is to make your own! Make your own? Yep, you read that right. Amazon, and several other stores online sell starter kits to make your own Kombucha. It is incredibly easy, saves you money, and allows you to control the sugar content in your food. I highly suggest you give it a whirl - your insides will thank you!

Carb Loading

*****A quick note before most of you get too excited. This specific type of carb loading is only for those who train extremely hard, do mud runs, or are professional athletes as it contains the ingestion of basically everything I told you already NOT to eat. It's a fascinating part of our physiology if you care to read however, if your goal is only extreme weight loss you may skip to the next section on protein****

This is a current method popularized by physicist John Kiefer and most of this information was written based off of his articles, or first book Carbnite. John grew up as a fat kid turned bodybuilder with a mean sweet tooth. Every bodybuilding competition he entered in he would mess up because he could not control his tendency for sugar. The next competition he signed up for he promised himself he would start early, be ahead of schedule, and stick to his nutrition plan. Eight weeks from getting on stage, he was walking by a donut shop and gave in. He sat down and ate over a dozen donuts. Demoralized, he went home and fell into a deep carbohydrate coma, and was prepared to face the consequences the next day. To his surprise he actually woke up and was LEANER than the day before. His muscles were full and he felt amazing. As a physicist he started researching like a mad man, and here is what he found.

No matter what you eat the night before, every human rises from their sleep burning fat. Breakfast, led by the mainstream media, and the carbohydrate industry, has us believe that it is the most important meal of the day. They hammer that down our throat every day on the radio, on T.V. and in the magazines of your choice. There's a problem though because cortisol (an adrenal hormone) levels naturally raise through the evening, continue as we sleep, and peak around wake-up time. Cortisol breaks down body tissue, which can include muscle, but only if certain signals in the body direct it to do so. The specific signal is elevated insulin levels and high cortisol levels (we spoke about this earlier). Having a high-carb breakfast (muffins, bagels, pancakes, cereal) will actually switch on the potential of the body to burn *muscle and store fat*!

If cortisol acts alone, in the absence of insulin, it forces the body to preferentially burn body fat; this is the exact scenario you find yourself upon waking, if you don't screw it up by eating that delicious waffle with strawberries and whipped cream. If you don't eat anything, or very little, cortisol continues signaling the release of body fat for metabolism, just as it did through the previous hours of sleep.

There is another nasty problem with high insulin levels plus high cortisol levels that many, many people do not know about. When insulin and cortisol are elevated together, the body gets another signal; start making as many new, empty fat cells as possible—the max number of which being determined by how much body fat you already have stored, the more fat, the more empty fat cells created (6). The new fat cells start off empty, which means the cells send out hormonal signals to slow metabolism, because empty fat cells have one goal, to get full. Once full, the cells last forever. Only after 10 years of being kept empty do these fat cells die through a process known as apoptosis (their guts spill out through the membrane, almost like getting turned inside out). There's a way we can speed up this fat-cell-destruction process and its called Carb Loading.

Carbohydrate metabolism isn't as simple or easy to understand as pop-media and even sports nutritionists imply. The classic version used to be that you eat sugar; carbs get into the bloodstream as sugar, which hits the pancreas and causes a release of insulin. Insulin rushes through the body and shuttles sugar into the cells it chooses. This is a very broad view of what actually happens.

As scientists researched things a bit closer, it's not insulin that carries sugar into cells; there are very specialized transporters that exist within each cell to bring sugar across the cell membrane, transporters called, not surprisingly, glucose transporters (GLUTs). There are 12 of these transporters in three classes. The class I GLUTs—GLUT1 through GLUT4—are the best understood. (There are two more classes that contain GLUTs 5-12, but—besides the fructose transporter, GLUT5—science is still deciphering their function, and some, like GLUT6 and GLUT8 actually block glucose transport, weird, I know.)

Different tissues in the body contain different transporters. Tissues with GLUT1s, GLUT2s or GLUT3s use sugar whether insulin levels rise or not. Cells of the pancreas, kidney, small blood vessels and nervous system, including those in the brain, contain GLUTs 1 through 3. That doesn't mean these cells need sugar, only that they can always use it regardless of the presence or absence of insulin.

GLUT4, however, sits tucked within the surface of the cell membrane until the cell senses insulin, at which point the GLUT4s move to the surface and start grabbing sugar and pulling it in. Fat cells and muscle cells contain GLUT4 receptors. When the experts say the body is most sensitive to insulin in the morning, they mean GLUT4 tissue—body fat and skeletal muscle.

There are two interesting facts about this information, one good, and one bad. The plus side to this information: fat cells can't store as much sugar as fat in the evening. The minus side: muscles can't use carbs as effectively either. There is, however, a way to keep the plus and eliminate the minus. It's something everybody reading this hopefully already does and it's called lifting weights! By beginning our workout sometime between 3-6:30pm we can optimize the effect lifting weights has on our GLUT 4 transporters and they essentially become hypersensitive to shuttling sugar into the muscle cell, and virtually shut off the signal to shuttle fat into the fat cell. This gives us our win-win situation that everyone is looking for. The key is resistance training. As you'll see with the performance guide, with the use of carb loading you can eat a tremendous amount of sugary carbohydrates like ice-cream, donuts, and cookies which will help you recover from your extreme training faster, gain muscle and lose weight in the process. You can still lift in the morning, and carb load in the evening, it will just not be OPTIMAL, and in all likelihood you will stay without sugary carbohydrates till the evening time like we discussed. In the same respect you can lift past 7pm and carb load, this also is not OPTIMAL, and we will not have as much time to eat as we probably need (6).

Now, some of you are thinking this is too good to be true. You're saying I can eat whatever I want after lifting and not get fat?!?! Where do all the extra calories go? Answer: They are burned off as heat. You will notice two things the night of your first carb load. The first is that you will sleep like a baby. The second is you will wake up in a puddle of your own sweat. What happens is that your body needs to burn off the excess calories by raising your body's own temperature and cook it internally. If this happens before you go to bed, you know you nailed the carb load! The enhanced recovery effects of this way of eating are monstrous! I mean think about it. How do you eat enough to recover from some of these challenging workouts without filling up your fat cells at the same time? Carb loading is how! A slight warning though, this is for high-level athletes looking for a true performance diet only. You cannot just eat whatever you want without taking advantage of exercising. If you are looking to decrease body fat and bodyweight, we will discuss the rapid fat loss guide below, as well as a maintenance guide. But first we need to discuss our last macronutrient, protein!

Chapter Two at a Glance:

- Your body requires zero carbohydrates to stay alive; athletes need them for performance.
- Stop eating or limit anything containing high fructose corn syrup.
- Hyper palatable/rewarding foods are foods containing fat, salt, and sugar, which tells your brain to tell you to eat excessively.
- Grains, especially whole grains contain toxins that create extremely deleterious conditions in our body and should be removed completely or highly limited.
- Fruits are not a health food; they are candy and should be extremely limited. Green papaya, banana, plantains, and mangoes have resistant starches that your good gut bacteria eat and thrive on.
- Milk has been linked to many autoimmune diseases and contains measurable amounts of pus. The sugar content is very high, and the protein it contains (casein) has been linked directly to cancer and other life-threatening diseases. A-2 milk is a better option, but not by much.
- Eat fermented foods daily, ideally with every meal.
- Carb loading is a great tool for athletes looking to recover faster from heavy exercise.

Chapter 3: Protein

"Eat right. Stay fit. Live long. Die quick."
~Liping Zhao

Protein quality refers, in a general sense, to how well or poorly the body will use a given protein. More technically, protein quality refers to how well the essential amino acid (EAA) profile of a protein matches the requirements of the body; the digestibility of the protein and of the amino acids (AAs) also plays a role. The pathways for protein digestion are actually very wasteful, this is what makes some protein supplements better than others, as their digestibility and ability of the body to use them (we call this bioavailability) varies. As you will see, not all proteins are created equal.

Sources of protein:

Animal Protein

Protein sources based on meat (beef, chicken, pork, fish, eggs) are your number one go to source of protein. Meat protein will contain about 7 grams of protein per ounce. So a 3 oz. piece of meat (about the size of a deck of cards) will generally have about 21-24 grams of dietary protein. The protein content of other foods depends on the food. One word of caution is red meat. Read meat contains a lot of iron in it. The human body is good at taking iron in, bad at getting iron out. Red meat consumption should be slightly limited because of this. The only exception is for women while they are menstruating. Since they are losing blood, and blood contains iron, it would be wise to consume red meat during that time to replenish it, especially if you are doing CrossFit or training at a very high state!

***********News Flash***********

HEALTH
OCT 26 2015, 8:46 AM ET

Ham, Sausages Cause Cancer; Red Meat Probably Does, Too, WHO Group Says

by MAGGIE FOX

As I am writing this book I have been attacked with questions about the recent study that emerged showing that red meat causes cancer. I eat a lot of meat and tell everyone else to as well. When the World Health Organization publishes a paper (Red meat causes cancer) placing red meat in the same category as asbestos, I can understand your cause for concern. I tell everyone there are three sides to every coin. There's true, there's false, and there's that cool ribbed side that no one seems to mention (unless you're a nickel or penny). Reading research is not just about reading the abstract (what they proved or believe to be true), or reading the conclusion (what they disproved or believe to be false) it’s about deciphering that cool little ribbed side in between. That's what we are going to do here.

The state of our food is in obvious disarray! With genetic modification, cows being fed grains, and a whole host of other things, eating can be down right scary sometimes. Let's get down to the issues of this study though:

- Research was gathered on 800 epidemiological studies
- Epidemiological means participants signed up for a study and then were given a questionnaire years later. This was not a controlled study!

- Researchers are saying processed red meat definitely causes cancer, and steak and hamburger "probably" cause cancer.

- It showed a relative risk of getting colorectal cancer to increase by 18%, which means a comparison between groups, where the absolute risk (the likelihood of it happening at all) was only at 1.8%.

- Researchers didn't differentiate between the QUALITIES of the meat being consumed.

- 50 grams or more a day of "processed" red meat is considered to be the increased risk number.

- The hemoglobin in bacon or hot dogs leads to DNA damage through N-Nitroso compounds.

- Heterocyclic Amines are a damaging compound found in the charred or blackened bits of food that are a contributing factor to cancer. Let's face it; sausages and bacon (processed meat) burn easier than a steak or hamburger.

- The iron in red meat is in a heme-form and is not as easily digestible as plant based iron in say kale or spinach that is more tightly bound and in a non-heme form. Iron from red meat may stay in the gut longer as a result and cause damage, thus the increase in colorectal cancer.

- Meat also contains an antigen called Neu5Gc. Antigens cause allergies, and this one actually causes people who are allergic to Neu5Gc to experience inflammation as a reaction to it (10). Inflammation is a carcinogen!

So how do we enjoy meat and NOT get cancer?

- Marinate your meat and use spices.

- Eat cruciferous (broccoli, cauliflower, etc.) vegetables or fruits (especially your green fruits!) with your meat to neutralize N-Nitroso compounds in processed red meat that create problems in the gut that can lead to cancer (9).

- Eat red meat with lots of fermented foods, probiotics, and lovely drinks like Kombucha.
- Don't burn your meat or use high heat to cook every day.

- Don't eat processed meat every day.
- Supplement with omega-3 fatty acids to stay balanced.

The bottom line is that anything in excess will kill you. Too much oxygen will make you pass out, and a lady died from drinking too much water during a contest to win a Nintendo Wii, her organs literally drowned. This study's headline is very misleading to the general consumer, but provides that great shock and awe attention grabbing title. It's misleading because the public only understands the headline, they take it for face value, when the truth in understanding is written on the side no one pays attention to.

If you remember form chapter 1, the typical American diet contains the poor ratio of bad to good fats at an astounding 20:1. This imbalanced ratio is what leads to excessive inflammation and all the cancer causing markers out there. Be conscious. Don't eat bacon and sausage every day, that's not what we advocate. When you do, eat raw vegetables or take digestive enzymes to aid in digestion and neutralize these alleged cancer-causing factors we just talked about and you'll be fine.

When it comes to meats, the greatest thing we need to have at the forefront of our mind is that whatever the animal you are eating ate, will become assimilated in your body when the protein and fat is digested. This makes animal protein a sneaky little transport vessel for lectins. If the beef and chicken you are eating is being fed soy and grains to fatten them up, you are now eating soy and grains as well. The makes verbiage such as grass fed AND finished, or pasture raised chicken very important. Here is how everything breaks down and what you want to look for when purchasing meat:

Beef – Beef needs to be grass fed and grass finished. If it does not say grass finished on the package or 100% grass fed, then it was finished in the slaughterhouse with a grain diet to fatten the cow up. The grains and soy being fed to the cows are not fit for human consumption and are thus fed to the cow. The grains upset the cow's stomachs because cows stomachs are not meant to digest grains and are thus fed antacids as well. But let's not stop there when we can get more disgusting….. Grain fed beef has enough antibiotics in it to kill bacteria in a petri dish! Remember what we said in chapter 2 about how antibiotics kill healthy cells as well as infected cells? Well the food you are eating to repair and replicate your cells now contains antibiotics that can kill your cells. Just say no to grain fed beef!

Chicken – if you thought chicken was harmless then think again. For a while now chicken has become a large part of the American diet and is dubbed by many to be healthier because of its leanness. The problem is if you look at all of the verbiage on the packaging once again it says fed an "All vegetarian diet." Chickens are insectivores and this all-vegetarian diet consisting of soy and grains goes against what the chicken naturally evolved on. Not only that, but chicken was found in a study to contain the most phthalates which is a synthetic compound that makes plastics softer. Researchers found that the more phthalates a pregnant woman consumed, the small her boys penis would be. A high concentration of phthalates in men also damages the DNA in his sperm. This stuff is not only making us feel sick or lethargic, it is also hitting us on an evolutionary level. Where we reproduce! Free-range chicken is a farce because the chickens can still be held in a crate. If the gate is open for 5 minutes a day, the producer can label their package "Free range." The only type of chicken (or eggs) you want to consume is pastured, or pasture raised. These chickens feed off the land and run around to their hearts delight doing what chickens do. Since gaining this knowledge I have reduced my chicken consumption to about twice per month and have noticed a huge difference in the way I feel. I suggest you do the same!

Lamb – There is not too much research I can gather on the dangers of lamb meat. The primary thing we need to be aware of is that lambs also eat a grass only diet. All lamb meat you eat as a result needs to be 100% grass fed and grass finished.

Pork – Same as above, pork needs to be pasture raised. The pigs need to be eating an indigenous diet and free to roam. Pigs are omnivores, so once again if a package is telling you it was fed an all-vegetarian diet, you can buy it if you want, but I suggest you use it as a Frisbee rather than for food. If you're into bacon, make sure it is uncured which means it is sans preservatives, which eliminates the nitrates and nitrites our cardiovascular system does not like. Pork belly is an amazing source of fat, especially in the morning.

Turkey – Due to it leanness once again, I really only consume turkey at thanksgiving. I find it to be dry and boring, but if it's one of your favorites all you need to look for is the pasture-raised label. This ensures it isn't fed complete trash.

Duck – one of my favorites that I feel in love with in Hawai'i was duck. When cooked properly, it is a most satiating meat! Duck fat contains a great mixture of omega-3 and omega-6 fatty acids and is amazing to cook with. Make sure to look for the pasture-raised label!

Fish and Shellfish – Avoid farm raised fish and shellfish at all costs. Not only are they fed soy, which you end up eating through eating them, but they swim around in much more polluted water. Fish filter pollutants with their gills, but shellfish on the other hand do not have that luxury so you end up eating a plethora of toxins with your food. This makes eating wild caught fish and shellfish a no brainer. With wild caught sea life, we need to be aware of mercury content. The Natural Resources Defense Council has compiled a list of fish with the least amount of mercury, to the highest, which you will want to check out in full. For now, here is a condensed version to get you started:

Least Mercury

- Anchovy
- Butterfish
- Catfish
- Clams
- Crabs

- Crawfish (try one from New Zealand!)
- Flounder
- Haddock
- Herring
- Mackerel
- Oysters
- Salmon
- Scallops
- Shrimp
- Whitefish

High Mercury (Avoid)

- Bluefish
- Grouper
- Halibut
- Marlin
- Sea bass (Chilean (I know, devastating))
- Shark
- Swordfish
- Tuna (Ahi)

I now eat fish or shellfish close to 3-4 times per night, and thoroughly enjoy doing so especially living in South Florida where I have access to it being very fresh. As I mentioned in chapter 1, fish contain omega-3 fatty acids, which boost our health beyond belief. Become a fish lover and you will love how you feel!

Cheeses:

Dairy products generally always contain some protein although the amounts can vary. A typical 8 oz. serving of cheese will contain about 12 grams of protein. We discussed the best types of cheeses to eat in the FATS section, please reference back if you need to. The fat content of dairy can vary significantly from zero in fat-free dairy (which you should never consume) to moderate levels in full-fat foods. I caution against anyone consuming fat-free cheese. I remember when I was younger and it first hit the shelves. My friend and I (whom were on the fat-free kick because we though it was healthier) bought some and tried making grilled cheese sandwiches. The cheese would not melt. It was disgusting, but we ate it anyway. The fat in cheese is solid at room temperature or below; it should melt when the temperature goes higher than that. This is NORMAL! Cheese, especially American cheese, is highly processed and should be avoided because of this.

Vegetable Protein

Beans and Nuts

For their caloric content, these guys tend to be lower in terms of protein, but are still a great source to have as a side dish. Beans generally contain a good bit of carbohydrate (along with a chunk of fiber), nuts contain a good bit of dietary fat as long as we are eating them raw and are following the guidelines we described in the fats section. The beans need to be cooked, and should be limited due to their lectin content – even after they are cooked. Stick to 1-4 handfuls of the nuts I recommended in the fat section per day. No cashews, or peanuts!

Vegetables

Veggies are a great source of protein if you are a vegan or vegetarian, but will not be the main source of protein for this guide. Yes, I know a 100 calories of broccoli has more protein in it than a 100 calories of red meat, but lets be honest on which one tastes better and is more satiating when cooked. When consuming vegetables (for protein or as a side dish) eat as many of the vegetables as you can raw. Raw vegetables contain enzymes like the ones we described in chapter 2 and aid in digestion. The amount of enzymes our body has to make is inversely related to the length of our life. The more raw food we consume, the less enzymes our body has to make, and the longer our life span will be.

To paint a clearer picture, let's take a quick time out and look a little closer at these little buddies. There are three types of Enzymes we need to be educated on:

- Metabolic enzymes catalyze, or spark, the reactions within the cells. Metabolic enzymes run the body's organs, tissues, and cells. Without them our bodies would not work. Among their chores are helping to turn phosphorus into bone, attaching iron to our red blood cells, healing wounds, thinking, and making our heart beat (7).

Kind of important!

- Digestive enzymes break down foods, allowing their nutrients to be absorbed into the bloodstream and used in body functions. Digestive enzymes ensure that we get the greatest possible nutritional value from foods (7).

- Food enzymes are enzymes supplied to us through the foods we eat. Nature has placed them there to aid in our digestion of foods. This way, we do not use as many of the body's "in-house" enzymes in the digestive process (7).

To show the effect enzymes can have on our health, scientists performed a study in which rats were fed enzyme free sugar. This resulted in a decrease in the size of the pituitary gland, which regulates growth, reproduction, and various other metabolic activities (5).

Constantly eating cooked food can not only decrease the size of your pituitary gland, but also create a situation in your gut called digestive leukocytosis. When this occurs, the immune system actually does not recognize the cooked food in the intestines and thinks it is foreign matter. White blood cells rush in ready to attack……… nothing. Have you ever gotten really tired after eating breakfast, lunch, or dinner? This is what is happening to you. Your body is making enzymes to digest the cooked food, which requires energy, and your immune system is in attack mode telling you to rest so it can get rid of your illness, although no illness exists. Consuming at least 10% of your food raw, before eating your cooked food stops leukocytosis dead in it's tracks. Here are some of the best organic veggies to eat raw:

Cabbage – Helps with and prevents stomach ulcers.

Celery – Helps with high blood pressure, has natural amounts of sodium, and helps with joint and urinary tract inflammation. Never eat wilted celery as it contains a very bad toxin.

Garlic, Onions, Leeks – Naturally antibiotic, anti-fungal, and anti-tumor.

Mushrooms – Anti inflammatory, anti - carcinogenic.

Soy Protein:

It is my suggestion that soy protein be heavily avoided or cut out all together. The issue with soy is most soy today contains something called phytoestrogens, and these phytoestrogens are estrogen mimickers in the body. If you're a male, and you're consuming extra estrogen it's going to give you more feminine characteristics. If you're a woman consuming foods that increase estrogen levels, it's going to increase your risk of breast cancer, cervical cancer, PCOS (polycystic ovary syndrome) and other hormone imbalance-related disorders.

Another big deal is that 90 percent (yep, 90!) of soy today is also genetically modified. **Genetically modified foods** are linked to many health problems because they kill off good bacteria in your gut, known to have a probiotic like benefit, and also damage the working of your digestive system. It's troubling to think that you have an entire line of food made up by science that flies off of the shelves in local supermarkets as long as you add a little sugar. To seal the deal, Google Monsanto if you've been living under a rock for the last 20 years, and see what the general media has to say about their structure as a company. To explain it here would take volumes and neither you nor I have that kind of time!

Protein Rules:

Typically the average person goes wrong in two different areas in regards to eating protein. The first is not eating a solid piece of protein at EVERY meal. Just because bok choy and pasta has protein in it does not mean that we are having a proper meal. The second is how much protein and what type. You should be mixing up your protein choices throughout the day in order to change the amino acid and lipid profile of the food you have at every meal. For instance, do not eat chicken with every meal, seven days a week.

Supplemental protein is a multi-billion dollar industry that for the large part has most of the population slurping down exotic sounding, delicious tasting shakes that can be ready in seconds, and gone even faster. The message we get from these companies is more, more, more. The product on the right says 52 grams of protein per serving, and the product on the left says 60 grams of protein so if I want more muscle, I'm going with the product on the left! Not so fast Arnold. Besides the fact that most of these protein drinks contain more fillers and toxins than protein, when it come to protein more is not always better. Why, you ask? Because of a little known term called nitrogen balance.

When you consume protein in the form of food or amino acid supplements, the body breaks it down and releases nitrogen. Nitrogen is then broken down further to release ammonia, urea, and uric acid, most of which is released in your urine. When the amount of protein we consume is less than what we used that day, we are in a negative balance or debt. This means we are in a catabolic or muscle wasting state. When the amount of protein we consume matches what we use, we are in balance.

However, when the amount of protein we consume is greater than the amount we use we are in a positive balance or what we term an anabolic (muscle building) state. This is good right? Well, maybe. If we keep this positive balance for too long, and if the nitrogen build up becomes too great, we run into trouble and may not even know it. People who exercise rigorously (walking is not exercise it is movement) don't have too much to worry about, but if you're not exercising and consuming 200g of protein a day, certain unfavorable metabolic responses start to take place.

First, everyone knows ammonia is a toxic compound and needs to be expunged by the body. When we get to around the 250g mark for protein consumption the kidney's get backed up and slow the elimination of ammonia, which stresses them out. In the process, this can cause dehydration because the kidneys need more water to process the ammonia and will start to pull it from other sources in the body if we are not drinking enough. Finally, a gene that researchers have found is directly correlated with accelerated aging called mTOR (mammalian target of rapamycin) is turned on by excessive caloric and amino acid consumption. Consuming less protein can actually lengthen your life span!

How much do we eat then? The US Recommended Dietary Allowance (RDA) is 0.36 grams of protein per pound of body weight per day (8). This is the number we use for our rapid fat loss guide. If you add exercise to the mix, this will help reduce body fat pretty quickly in the process. So if you are a female weighing 130lbs, here is your calculation:

130lbs x .36 = 46.8.

- If you have 3 meals, then you're looking at roughly 16 grams of protein per meal.
- For those of you looking to maintain your muscle mass we want to consume about .55 grams of protein per pound of bodyweight. Here are the calculations for a 175lb male:

175lbs x .55 = 96.25.

- If you were eating 3 meals, then you would be consuming 32 grams of protein per meal, or roughly one large chicken breast.
- Lastly, for all you out there trying to add muscle to your frame, we want to eat about .7 grams of protein per pound of bodyweight. Here is what it looks like for a 195lb male:

195lbs x .7 = 136.5 grams per day.

- Split into three meals he would be consuming 45.5 grams of protein per meal.

There you have it guys. I've been in the super-athlete world long enough. I've worked with pro football players, triathletes, and MMA fighters that consume up to 2 grams of protein per pound of bodyweight. It's just too much, and when I advise them to consume less, they always end up feeling better! The protein supplement we recommend contains only 10g of protein per scoop because that's all you need! For a really tough workout you can use 20g, no problem, but the companies selling you jugs of protein with 60g per scoop are absolutely insane! Don't go for it and save your money, most of that powder is going right into the toilet anyway.

Water

When people ask me what they should drink, my answer is always water! I don't use pre-work out drinks and Gatorade and PowerAde contain too much sugar to be used during exercise! Water is an amazing substance. It is the only non-polluting, sustainable source of energy that suspends all of the problems caused by fossil fuels, explosives, and fires. We can run everything on the ground on hydro-electricity. We can make fuel by using some of this electricity to split water into hydrogen and oxygen. We can store water and irrigate dry places to make them green. Water is necessary for growing food, and allowing green plants to turn carbon dioxide back into oxygen. Water is therefore necessary for hunger, thirst, and breath. We should be amazed by water, instead we waste, and waste, and waste, and waste.

According to Dr. Mercola there are 6 different types of water available to us now. They are:

- **Purified water**: Water that is physically processed to remove impurities (e.g., distillation, deionization, reverse osmosis, carbon filtration, etc.)

- **Distilled water**: Water that is boiled and evaporated away from its dissolved minerals, and then the vapor is condensed.

- **Bottled Water**. This water is typically from a spring or has gone through reverse osmosis before it is bottled. However, some brands are simply bottled tap water that may or may not have gone through any additional filtering.

- **Alkaline water**: Water that has been separated into alkaline and acid fractions using electrolysis, which takes advantage of the naturally occurring electric charges found in the magnesium and calcium ions; in the drinking water industry.

- **Deionized or demineralized water**: Water in which the mineral ions (salts such as sodium, calcium, iron, copper, chloride and bromide) have been removed by exposing it to electrically charged resins that attract and bind to the salts.
- **Hard and soft water**: Hard water is any water containing an appreciable quantity of dissolved minerals; soft water is treated water in which the only cation (positively charged ion) is sodium (13).

Many people think water is boring and end up reaching for sugary additives, or zero calorie sweeteners. These are both trash! You're putting more chemicals along with food dyes into the water. What I do to spruce up my water is either put lemon in it, or I'll put a dash of Bragg's apple cider vinegar in there and it actually makes it taste sweet. Experiment with the amount so it's not overpowering and you will never go back to just regular ice water again!

But Chris, you're not drinking water out of the tap are you? I sure am.

Most people believe that tap water is dangerous due to the chemicals that are put in our water supply by our local officials, and they are somewhat correct. The problem is that these same people think that bottled water is much safer, and here is where they are completely wrong.

In a documentary called ***Tapped*** we learn the shocking truth about bottled water and the carcinogens it contains, yes I said carcinogens as in cancer causing agents. Here is a quick recap of the information provided in the documentary:

- By 2030 we will lack enough safe drinking water for some parts of the world.

- Companies extract water for free and sell it to us at a ridiculous mark up.

- Bottles marked PETE or PET contains plastic made from crude oil. The chemicals leak into the water and then we drink it.

- Bottled water companies test their own water, and do **NOT** have to report their findings. Many independent tests have found a wide variety of poisonous chemicals in bottled water.

- Some bottled water like Dasani, is just filtered tap water.

- Bottled water accounts for 1.5 million tons of waste per year; some ends up in streams, and the ocean.

Basically, when it comes down to it, we are buying tap water at a 3000% mark up. I don't know anyone that has the money to spend that much more on any product, anywhere. The other scary fact we learn in the film is that when heated, the chemicals in the water leach into the plastic. This correlates with a study published in Environmental Health Perspectives that even plastics that do not contain the toxin BPA are still releasing estrogen like hormones into our food and drink (14).

With this knowledge, I recommend that NOBODY drink bottled water. Voss, Perrier, and other manufacturers that use glass bottles are better options, but still there is no regulation on what is in the water! What do we drink when we are thirsty then?

I have been waiting over 10 years for this solution to arise. I've known that the Brita water filters, or those similar to Brita make the water taste better, but are very poor at removing anything harmful found in the water. Enter AquaTru Water Filter. AquaTru is your best bet for PURE drinking water and guess what? You use your own tap water. Not only that, but there is no installation required, the filters last for 2-3 years, and when you have to replace them, they are cheap and easy to install.

Ultimately it is your call though. You can think that all these claims the movie is making are not really as bad as they are saying. You can choose to think I am recommending a product to get a commission. Whatever the case, facts are facts. Water and only water should be going into your body and I feel the AquaTru is the best. I have been using one for two months now as I'm writing this and there is a noticable difference in the way the water tastes, and how I feel. My coffee even tastes better since I've been using the AquaTru water. Check out the AquaTru, you will not be disappointed!

Supplements

While you may not find the need for most of these supplements, not all supplements are created equal. Rest assured, if I'm recommending a product, it has been tested by me at length and the purity and quality are as high as we can get. Most of these can be found on Amazon.com and is the only platform I use to purchase my supplements.

Muscle Shake

The best mixable protein supplement on the market. Made from 100% New Zealand grass-fed Beef.

- No protein spiking ingredients like creatine, glycine, hydrolyzed gelatin, or taurine.
- No soy protein or rice protein.
- All hydrolyzed beef protein, pre digested protein.
- The best tasting protein powder ever!

Sports Research Vitamin D

Supplementing with 5-15,000IU of vitamin D per day is crucial for the absorption and metabolism of calcium and phosphorous, which have various functions, especially the maintenance of healthy bones. Here are some other really amazing reasons to supplement with vitamin D every day:

- Aids the immune system - vitamin D may be an important way to arm the immune system against disorders like the common cold, say scientists from the University of Colorado Denver School of Medicine, Massachusetts General Hospital and Children's Hospital Boston.

- MS risk - it may reduce the risk of developing multiple sclerosis. Multiple sclerosis is much less common the nearer you get to the tropics, where there is much more sunlight, according to Dennis Bourdette, chairman of the Department of Neurology and director of the Multiple Sclerosis and Neuroimmunology Center at Oregon Health and Science University, USA.

- Maintaining cognitive functions - vitamin D may play a key role in helping the brain keep working well in later life, according to a study of 3000 European men between the ages of 40 and 79.

- Healthy body weight - vitamin D probably plays an important role in maintaining a healthy body weight, according to research carried out at the Medical College of Georgia, USA.

- Asthma symptoms and frequency - it can reduce the severity and frequency of asthma symptoms, and also the likelihood of hospitalizations due to asthma, researchers from Harvard Medical School found after monitoring 616 children in Costa Rica.

- Rheumatoid arthritis - it has been shown to reduce the risk of developing rheumatoid arthritis in women.

- Protects from radiation damage - a form of vitamin D could be one of our body's main protections against damage from low levels of radiation, say radiological experts from the New York City Department of Health and Mental Hygiene.

- Vitamin D and cancer risk - various studies have shown that people with adequate levels of vitamin D have a significantly lower risk of developing cancer, compared to those whose levels are low. Vitamin D deficiency was found to be prevalent in cancer patients regardless of nutritional status in a study carried out by the Cancer Treatment Centers of America.

- T.B. recovery - high vitamin D doses can help people recover from tuberculosis more rapidly, researchers reported in September 2012 in the *Proceeding of the National Academy of Sciences (PNAS)*.

- Heart attack risk - a study published in September 2012 suggested that low levels of vitamin D might increase the risk of heart attack and early death.

Braggs Apple Cider Vinegar

Bragg's has been an amazing addition to my health for over 10 years now. It is a fermented food and thus contributes greatly to the internal workings of our body by letting the good gut bacteria thrive, killing off the bad gut bacteria. I used to get sick 2-4 times per year before I started taking a small sip of this magical potion before bed. I have since been cold free and when I do start to feel a bit of a scratchy throat, I run to take a sip. It has never let me down! Here is just a little of what it does:

- Rich in enzymes & potassium.
- Support a healthy immune system.
- Helps control weight.
- Promotes digestion & ph Balance.
- Helps soothe dry throat.
- Helps remove body sludge toxins.
- Helps Maintain healthy skin.

MediHerb M1050 Adrenal Complex

Take 1-3 pills per day, and you may want to check with a doctor before you take it. Fatigued adrenals can lead to a host of different issues in the body. A weakened immune system, restless nights of sleep, reduced recovery from exercise, just to name a few. Here are the benefits of this supplement:

- Restore adrenal function to reduce the effects of stress on the body
- Support adrenal gland health and energy production to help combat fatigue

- Help the body adapt to the challenges of everyday life
- Promote the body's normal resistance function
- Support a healthy immune system when experiencing occasional stress

Bulletproof Upgraded Coffee

Upgraded coffee is the only type of coffee I consume anymore. It's made and tested for toxins by Dave Asprey, the founder of Bulletproof Coffee. The harsh fact about it is that the USA does not have any regulations regarding mold toxins in our coffee so we get the worlds leftovers. In a recent finding, it was reported that over 91% of coffee beans from Brazil had dangerous mold toxins. If you are crashing hard after drinking your coffee or you're not getting the kick you normally do, then your coffee is moldy, and this is for you. Hell, everyone should be drinking this coffee everywhere it is that pure.

Bulletproof Brain Octane Oil/XCT Oil

Brain octane oil is again from the brain of Dave Asprey. It is pure, super concentrated coconut oil and it does a bunch of great things for our brain and gut. It balances out yeast in the small intestine and give us a laser like focus. The benefits of coconut oil reach from pulling toxins out of the body, to actually slowing down the symptoms of Alzheimer's disease! I put two tablespoons in my coffee every morning.

Digestive Enzymes – Rainbow Light

For better digestion: Take one pill with every meal containing mostly cooked food. Many modern health researchers believe that on the same scale as our need for air and water, enzymes play equally crucial roles in enabling proper cellular and bodily health and function.

Remember we said your length of life is inverse to the amount of enzymes your body has to produce! Most people properly associate enzymes with supporting healthy digestive function, however there are actually many different classes of enzymes; digestive, anti-inflammatory and antioxidant, just to name a few. Our bodies need a broad spectrum and replenishment of them at all times.

For better recover from exercise: Take between 5-15 enzymes on an empty stomach first thing in the morning. Enzymes are required for just about every healthy process in your body, but are especially important for digestion, absorption & regulating dangerous inflammation. Taking a large amount of enzymes on an empty stomach leaves the enzymes with no work to do in the stomach or small intestine so they enter the blood stream and start to help repair muscle tissue by eliminating inflammation. Here's a quick snippet from a piece titled "How to use enzymes for exercise" written by one of my favorite exercise guru's Ben Greenfield:

- In an Annals of The NY Academy Of Science article found in the excellent book "Enzymes & Enzyme Therapy," author Anthony Cichoke highlights how recovery from sprains and strains can decrease from eight weeks of inactivity to an impressive two weeks of inactivity with the consumption of enzymes.

- Another study entitled "Protease supplementation improves muscle function after eccentric exercise" looked into the use of protease supplementation to reduce the damaging effects of eccentric exercise and accelerate recovery of muscle function, possibly by regulating inflammation.
- In this study, subjects performed weight training via extension/flexion of the quadriceps muscle group. They were randomly assigned to consume 5.83 g daily of either a cellulose placebo or a proteolytic supplement containing fungal proteases, bromelain, and papain. They trained for 21 days. After the supplementation period, subjects donated blood samples before performing a 45-min downhill treadmill protocol at 60% of VO2max. Significant group differences were observed for peak torque at flexion, indicating higher force production in the protease group.
- In another study entitled "Effects of a protease supplement on eccentric exercise-induced markers of delayed-onset muscle soreness and muscle damage," researchers examined the effects of a protease supplement on selected markers of muscle damage and delayed-onset muscle soreness (DOMS). The

study used a double-blinded, placebo-controlled, crossover design. Twenty men were randomly assigned to either an enzyme supplement group or a placebo group.

- All subjects were tested for unilateral isometric forearm flexion strength, hanging joint angle, relaxed arm circumference, subjective pain rating, and plasma creatine kinase activity and myoglobin concentration. During these tests, the subjects in the supplement group ingested a protease supplement and subjects in the placebo group took microcrystalline cellulose. After testing and 2 weeks of rest, the subjects were crossed over into the opposite group and performed the same tests as during their first visits, but with the opposite limb.
- Overall, isometric forearm flexion strength was much greater (7.6%) for the supplement group than for the placebo group. These findings provided initial evidence that the protease supplement may be useful for reducing strength loss immediately after eccentric exercise and for aiding in short-term strength recovery.
- Perhaps even more impressive was the study "Double-Blind Clinical Study Using Certain Proteolytic Enzymes Mixtures In Karate Fighters," which was published in Enzymes Enzyme Therapy and showed mind blowing improvements after the use of digestive

enzymes for athletic injuries and subsequent recovery, including:

-Hematoma: recovery time decreased from 15.6 days to 6.6 days

-Swelling: recovery time decreased from 10 days to 4 days

-Restriction of movement: recovery time decreased from 12.6 days to 5 days

-Inflammation: recovery time decreased from 10.5 days to 3.8 days

-Unfit for training: recovery time decreased from 10.2 days to 4.2 days

- In the study "Therapy Of Ankles Join Distortions With Hydrolytic Enzymes; Results Of Double-Blind Clinical Trials", Dr. Baumuller used enzymes in a double blind study for ankle related injuries and found people could recover up to 50% faster.
- In another study entitled "Traumatic Injury In Athletes," in the International Rec. Medicine, Dr. Lichtmann treated boxers and found that with the use of enzymes, he could drop black eyes from 10 to 14 days of recovery to 1 to 3 days.

On the morning directly after a heavy workout, I will take up to 15 enzymes first thing in the morning on an empty stomach and have noticed a pretty dramatic decrease in recovery time. I have less soreness and that days training session is completed with greater ease.

Curcumin With Bioperine

Take 1200-3000 mg per day. Scientific studies are still underway, but Curcumin, is quickly becoming a sort of "magic bullet" supplement. Studies are showing it can help to significantly reduce arthritis/joint pain, boost brain function, reduce the risk of heart disease, alleviate digestive problems, prevent (and in some cases kill) cancer cell formation, and more.

Curcumin comes from turmeric, the yellow pigment in most Indian dishes. Simply consuming as much Indian food as possible does not work though because turmeric contains only about 5% curcuminoids for your body to use. For it to be effective we need about 1,200 mg per day.

Curcumin With Out Bioperine

Bioperine is a compound found in black pepper that enhances the absorption of curcumin. If you have a sensitivity to pepper, you may want to try this alternative as some people have reported having acid reflux while taking curcumin with Bioperine.

Udo's Oil

Take 1-2 tablespoons per day with a meal. Udo's oil is one of the most amazing supplements I have ever taken. I use it to maintain my balance of omega 3 fatty acids to omega 6 & 9 fatty acids. The benefits are, but not limited to:

- Improved Stamina And Endurance.

- Decrease Recovery Time And Soreness After Exercise And Competition And Speed The Healing Of Injuries.

- Improved Protein And Amino Acid Utilization To Help Build And Maintain Lean Mass.

- Decrease Fat Storage And Production And Support A Good Metabolic Rate.

- Improved Oxygen Uptake And Utilization.

- Optimize Glandular Function.

- Decreases Mild Joint Pain And Strengthen bones.

- Improve Circulation And Immune Function.

- Promotes Sleep, Elevates Mood, And Heightens reflexes.

Canned Coconut Milk

Coconut milk in the can is an amazing resource to help replace dairy, especially if you use a lot in your coffee like I do. The coconut milk in the bottles that the supermarkets sell has too many fillers, too much sugar, or not enough fat. Canned coconut basically goes from the tree into the can and is absolutely delicious on anything. I have a subscription on Amazon where I get a case sent to my home every month and it works out perfect for me. Some of the best brands are:

- Native Forest
- Thai Kitchen
- Goya
- Trader Joe's Organic

If you want to avoid guar gum additives and preservatives then Trader Joe's organic is the best option.

Magnesium

Several studies are now showing that over 80% of Americans are living their day-to-day lives with magnesium deficiency. So what you say? Well more than 50 serious health conditions are related to not having enough magnesium to go around when your cells need it. Not only does every organ in your body use magnesium, but it also helps promote:

- Nerve Function
- Cardiac activity
- Blood pressure regulation
- Hormonal interactions (Which can cause you to crave quick energy a.k.a. sugar!)
- Bone health

- Proper synthesis of proteins, fats, and nucleic acids (DNA).

In early 2015 I started supplementing with oral magnesium. Big mistake! I thought that more was better, and I got a serious case of disaster pants (diarrhea). On a positive note, it did prevent me from tossing and turning as much as I used to, but it was short lived, and on I went trying other supplements out.

The next form of magnesium I tried was Ancient Minerals spray. It worked really well, but because it was in oil form, rather than pill form, it made me and my clients itch really badly. Luckily I was listening to a podcast shortly after that and the guest was Ian Clark. Being extremely overweight, Ian was diagnosed with over 5 life threatening diseases including cancer and the doctor told him he would be dead in three months unless he started chemotherapy. Ian decided chemo wasn't for him and instead turned to playing Web MD to find out why these diseases developed in the first place. Long story short, he cured himself of said diseases, and in the process developed some really great products. Ease magnesium is one of those really great products.

Ease magnesium is a non-itching spray you can literally bathe in with no negative side effect. I have experienced a huge improvement in my sleep quality, a huge reduction in joint stiffness, and I also feel much more calm, and clear headed throughout the day. It is a staple in my nutrition supplement program and it should be in yours too. The main reason this spray is so effective is because your skin actually regulates the amount of magnesium your body can absorb. This means lather on as much as you want – no disaster pants here! It is available on his website activationproducts.com, or on amazon for a paltry $39. One bottle last me close to 4 months.

Chapter 3 At a Glance

- Red meat will NOT cause cancer.
- Any meat consumed must be fed an indigenous diet.
- Avoid chicken for the most part; eggs are OK as long as they are pasture raised.
- Fish and shellfish must be wild caught. Watch the mercury!
- Most vegetable protein is a great source. Be careful of lectin containing foods!
- Eating vegetables raw supply you with coveted enzymes that lighten the load on your digestive system.
- Too much protein can be hard on the kidneys and shorten your life span
- Drink filtered tap water, be wary of bottled water. The best filter is AquaTru.
- The supplements provided have been tried and true for many years and can boost your health due to their lack in our food supply.

Chapter 4: The Guides

"If you don't know where you're going, any road will take you there." ~Mark Twain

Training Your Digestive System

Picture the following scenario:

Imagine you go out one night for a nice brisk walk. The air is cool and the sky is clear. Off in the distance you hear barking and whining. As you get closer, you see a stray dog that got its collar stuck on a fence. No owner is around, and you happen to be an animal lover, so you free little cuddles and bring him home with you for the night. You go to sleep and when you wake up the dog has torn apart the house. Ripped pillows everywhere, furniture damaged, I bet you would think twice before you brought home another stray dog, right? Now what if you took that dog to a trainer? You could rest assured that when you woke up, your home would be intact.

The reason why I'm telling you this is because you need to think of your digestive system as your home in the previous story, and then think of the food you eat as the dog. When starting any one of the following diets, what you need to do is "train" your digestive system to adapt to what you are eating.

You need to eat the same things at the same time of day for several weeks, and in some cases months until your digestive system and endocrine system regulate. If you keep eating whatever you want to eat, whenever you want to eat it, this is what wreaks havoc in your body. Insulin is up one second, down the next. One minute you're happy, the next minute you're sad, and then an hour later you have uncontrollable anxiety. You need to train your digestive system like a dog. Tell it when to sit, stay, fetch, rollover; you need to control **it**, rather than **it** controlling **you**. I find in most cases this takes about 10-14 days, and it is between that time that I always lose someone. They come to me on day 10 and tell me about the headache, lack of energy, the sweet cravings and what not. I tell them to last just 4 more days and their whole life will change. Then I hear from them two days later and they said they got drunk and had taco bell with 4 churros. Anyone who makes it past that 14-day mark has always gone on to tremendous success no matter what.

Without any further banter, here are the last three guides you'll need for the rest of your life.

- A High-Speed Fat Loss Guide
- A Maintenance Guide
- A Performance Guide

The high-speed fat loss guide is obviously going to be the most challenging, and the performance guide is the maintenance guide turbo charged! The way these guides work is through what we call an allowable food list which makes things very simple. Whatever is on the list you can eat as much of as you want. Whatever is not on the list you cannot eat at all. Now, I know what you're thinking. How can I eat as much food as I want and still lose weight, or fat? The method is simple in the fact that these guides are nutrient restrictive, not calorie restrictive. There's no weighing food, or counting calories. What I find is when you limit calories, people tend to eat most of them too early in the day. Then 8pm comes around and they are ravenous! How do you expect to sleep being so hungry? With an allowable food list you can eat whatever you want at whatever time you want **AS LONG AS IT IS ON THE LIST!**

Sorry for yelling at you there. The reason why it is ok is because you will not be able to eat enough of the food on the list to gain weight. It's a non-factor. I mean have you ever heard of someone getting fat eating too much salmon and celery? No way Jose. The thing about real food is our body knows how to process it and use it for energy, or get rid of what cannot be used. When we eat processed food that contains chemicals and elements not found in nature, our body can't process them so they get stored which makes our body toxic and thus we gain weight!

Postprandial Period

A note for all of you really, really busy people out there. Number one, stop eating out so much and using busy-ness as an excuse. I used to work three jobs and still found time to cook all of my meals for the week. This is because I make nutrition a priority, not an afterthought. Number two; try to make it a point to relax after your meal. Postprandial refers to the two-hour mark after a meal where your food is digesting, hormones are elevating, nitric oxide is decreasing, and most of your blood is being drawn in towards the gut away from the muscles. I know it sounds impossible, but after we eat a meal, we should really lie down and rest, or kick back and do some reading. When I worked construction I would eat my lunch as quickly as I could everyday, then take a 30-45min nap until my lunch break was up. I know this sounds impossible, but cardiovascular disease is being linked to this postprandial period.

When you eat a meal and do stressful, or physical activity right after it puts a strain on the heart and doesn't allow the digestive system to do what it is supposed to do. It takes about two hours and 40 minutes for the stomach to empty a liquid meal (think protein shake), and 4 hours for the stomach to empty a solid meal. I've had people quit right in the middle of a workout before because they ate an hour or two before! Their body would not let them exercise due to the fact that it was digesting their food for them. I wait at least 3-4 hours after eating to exercise, and always rest 30-45 minutes after eating to avoid any problems, do your heart the same favor!

Why Coffee Is a Staple In Every Nutrition Guide

Coffee has been the target of ruthless misinformation campaigns for a very, very long time. I can remember a friend I had in high school who would jump on the bus with a cup of coffee every day. The kid was incredibly hyper and his energy persisted the entire day. I always used to think that was bad for you, but with the right information, things change.

Coffee has so many nutrients and antioxidants in it that it should be labeled and sold as a "superfood." When parents serve their overweight children fruit juice, soda, or sugar filled milk for breakfast and I tell them to stop, they ask what do I give my child then? When I tell them "coffee" I get this look of absolute horror as if I'm crazy, but my buddy from high school was on to something.

Coffee has been shown to improve memory recall, focus, and performance. Other studies show it lowers the risk of stroke and diabetes (12). Coffee has amazing thermogenic (fat burning) properties, and the polyphenols it contains feed good gut bacteria. It also decreases hunger by regulating insulin. This is why when we drink it; it makes us feel so darn good! I caution though, too much of a good thing can turn bad. I drink only one cup per day in the morning, and I recommend maximum two if you have a long day and want to train or need energy well past 5pm. Having 6 cups a day means you're dependent on something other than food to give you energy and this is unhealthy. Anyone with a caffeine headache can tell you that down regulating your caffeine receptors is not a fun process. Stick to 1-2 cups of Upgraded Coffee a day and you'll be fine.

If you have not had a cup of Dave Asprey's Bulletproof Coffee yet **you have not lived!** Dave was the CEO of a big firm in Silicon Valley by the age of 26. He was a millionaire, but he was fat. Six foot four, three hundred pounds fat. All of the diet and exercise regimes his doctors recommended and he tried failed to help him lose weight, or when it did, he couldn't keep it off. So Dave spent nearly $50,000 of his own money doing DNA and life hack testing on his own body. He was traveling in Asia when he was given a cup of coffee with Yak butter in it and it kept him going for hours!

Interested, he came back to the United States and started to experiment putting different butters in his coffee and found that grass fed butter was the main ingredient that has been missing in his diet his whole life. Weirdly enough, he still felt a crash on some days after finishing his coffee so he started to test the coffee he was drinking for mold toxins and opened up Pandora's box on himself.

Dave found out that when coffee is picked it often sits outside in the elements. The rain and sun eventually create mold and often times when the coffee is not roasted properly, the mold (mycotoxins) gets passed on to the consumer. Are you drinking 6 cups of coffee a day and still feeling like crap? That's because you're drinking toxic coffee! You may as well be drinking 6 beers every day, or taking 6 shots! These toxins back up in our system, stress it out and end up making us tired (the crash you feel when the caffeine wears off). Dave went to work and now has a company that grows coffee in Guatemala, roasts it to perfection, and tests it for toxins before it is shipped to your door.

The difference is undeniable! I have yet to crash or feel an energy drain from drinking bulletproof coffee. The first time I drank it, I wasn't hungry for 6 hours. Talk about controlling insulin!

Think about it. Who doesn't want to wake up, have a delicious cup of coffee, and then have a steady amount of energy for work all while not reaching for a snack every two hours that just teaches our body to store fat? The key is, like I said before, to blend 2 tablespoons of grass fed butter into your coffee every morning. It comes out as a delicious latte minus the 120 grams of sugar you get at staryucks.

When we eat grass fed butter, or grass fed beef, we get the proper micronutrients in the food that the cow gets by eating the grass. Cows did not evolve eating grains and left over garbage, so grain fed cows have less (astronomically less) nutrients in their meat and milk to satiate us. The absence of the grass makes their fat profile much different and less healthy as well, and this is where a lot of these "Red meat will kill you" studies come from. I have never seen a study bashing red meat that stated the quality of the meat was controlled to grass fed only. If you read the studies, it's usually the worst type of processed meat they can find like bacon, or sausage. Dave Asprey has been very vocal about wanting to live to 180 years old, and he's a huge grass fed meat promoter. Do you think he would be eating grass fed beef if it were really that terrible for you? In the words of Kevin McCalister, "I don't think so." I've said it 100 times already, but it's worth repeating; if you're going to eat red meat, make sure it says grass fed & finished on the package because some farmer's grass feed their cows, then grain feed them right before slaughter. It would be in your best interest to avoid grain fed beef all together.

You'll see in the guide tables that I have food recommended for breakfast, even though I do not personally eat breakfast on most days. I have my bulletproof coffee, and my first meal is between 12-2pm (I'm up at 5am). Some people may not be able to give breakfast up, or just plain don't like coffee. That's fine, you can also mix the butter, coconut oil, and collagen with tea if you like it, or just do what you enjoy. You'll see in the breakfast options I keep the carbs low (read no sugar), and the fat high, which is what you want in regards to keeping insulin at bay where it cannot signal new fat cells to be made. For those of you going the coffee route, you'll love the ease of making the coffee in the morning, and not having to pack extra food or worry about being hungry for snacks. The grass fed butter and brain octane keep you that full.

Preparing your food

While eating as much of your food, especially vegetables raw is ideal, it is not practical for most people, especially athletes. I try to eat as many raw vegetables during the day, and mostly cooked veggies at night because this allows me maintain my weight. Like I said earlier, raw food, especially vegetables contain a lot of natural enzymes, which means the fewer enzymes our body has to produce in order to digest our food, and the longer we will live. The caveat is that you will lose a lot of weight because it is more easily digested. I notice I feel great when eating raw foods, and that is why I primarily eat them throughout the day, but I feel more satiated with cooked food, and after a long day of work, that is why I eat mostly cooked food at night. Cooking food also has certain caveats we need to be aware of as well. Having said that, here are my rules for preparing my cooked foods.

Baking

I bake all of my chicken thighs, pork loins, and once in awhile, Salmon. I used to bake them somewhere around 350 degrees, but they would always turn out like cardboard. When I couldn't take it anymore, I finally did some research on how to properly bake chicken and found that high heat retains more juice than low heat and WOW, what a difference. I now bake all of the above meats at 425 degrees for between 15-22 minutes depending on the thickness of the cut of meat. Even if I leave it in a bit too long, then meat has never come out dry. I will also sometimes bake asparagus, with garlic and brussel sprouts along with my meat, and then add oil and salt when I take it out. Remember, if we can avoid heating our oils, do it!

Lightly Heated

My stovetop has the numbers 1-10 on it 10 being the hottest. I pan fry all of my hamburgers, steaks, lamb chops, and eggs between 3-4. Does it take longer?

SURE! But I never burn my meat and in some cases I don't even have to use oil. When I make hamburgers out of grass fed and finished beef, I put them in the pan before I turn the heat on. When I turn the heat on, the beef heats up slowly and the fats begin to creep out acting as natural grease. Also, because the heat is so low, the beef doesn't burn and the fats don't oxidize as badly creating inflammation in our body. Anytime I'm pan-frying I cook it medium rare, which leaves more enzymes in it, and also makes the beef taste better in my opinion. If I do need an anti-sticking agent, I'll use coconut oil, which makes the meat taste even more amazing, or a quick spread of grass-fed butter, which makes the beef taste richer. I can remember the first time I had used butter in the pan to make scrambled eggs; I was in heaven with how different they tasted compared to using non-stick cooking sprays. Yes it may be easier, but those chemicals are nasty!

Another word of caution would be to only use stainless steel or cast iron cookware. Do not use the non-stick pans! They contain a very nasty chemical that leeches into your food when heated. An easy experiment is to leave the pan on the stove with nothing in it and once it heats up you can smell the chemicals cooking and see a vapor coming off the pan. I have been using cast iron for years now and yes, again, it requires a bit of elbow grease at clean up, and you need to butter or oil it up before you use it, but there is no compromise for my health, and neither should there be for yours!

Boiled or Poached

When I do eat at a restaurant, which is rare, I always order my eggs poached. Studies have shown if you heat the yolk too much, you destroy the good fat and cholesterol in it, but poaching does not do this due to the sensitive nature of the boiling water cooking the food, and not the heat of the pan. I tried poaching eggs once myself and it was a disaster. I'm down to eating eggs once or twice a week, so it's no big deal, but I do enjoy them a lot more when poached as compared to scrambled.

I boil and drain the water in the following vegetables due to the dangerous toxins they contain:

- Kale
- Spinach
- Broccoli
- Beans
- Cauliflower

These vegetables contain a natural defense mechanism, which are toxic to our body when consumed raw. The full explanation is beyond the scope of this guide, but include aflatoxins, goitrogens, lectins (which we already discussed) and oxalates. Google them. It's pretty nasty stuff!

Throw Out Your Microwave

The first microwave was created in 1945, was 6 feet tall, and weighed around 750 pounds. Crazy right? Things get even crazier.

The microwave heats our food by sending waves of electrical and magnetic energy into the food, heating it from the inside out. Ever put something in a microwave too long and it explodes leaving a nice mess to clean up? Me too. The problem with this is that people want to assume these "micro-waves" are harmless, but Hans Hertel found them to be anything but.

Hans and some fellow scientist locked themselves in a hotel room in the early 1980's and did an experiment. They drank raw milk, and ate vegetables cooked a couple of different ways, and then they took blood samples at select periods after eating. What they found was disturbing.

When they drank the raw milk heated in the microwave, and ate the vegetables heated in the microwave, blood tests showed

- Decreased hemoglobin (which means less oxygen gets transported in the blood).
- HDL and LDL (good and bad cholesterol) both dropped.
- White blood cells counts decreased.

- There were signs of digestive leukocytosis (signs of poisoning and cell damage).

None of these markers showed up when food was heated with conventional methods (read: stove).

In April of 1992 the Journal of Pediatrics released a study showing if you microwave breast milk you destroy important disease fighting capabilities in the milk that need to get passed on to the child.

There have been many peer-reviewed studies on microwaved food showing:

- Asparagus lost 97% of its nutrients when microwaved.

- Also caused a reduction in Vitamin C.

- It renders allinase inactive in garlic which helps fight cancer.

- Degrades protein in milk, and meat.

- Alters amino acids in food, which becomes poisonous to the kidneys.

If you check the Internet, there are many opinion articles that say microwaves are just fine and dandy. There are also many scientific articles on the microwave advising against its use. Ultimately it is your decision, but I have lived without a microwave for 8 years now and have enjoyed nothing but good health. If you suffer from any of the following, I suggest you evaluate your microwave usage:

- Insomnia, night sweats.
- Frequent headaches, or dizziness.
- Swollen lymph nodes, or weak immune system.
- Impaired cognition.
- Depression, or irritability.
- Nausea, or appetite loss.
- Vision or eye problems.

The only benefit to using a microwave is convenience. If you're still on the fence then ask yourself this question: Why does your food blow up in the microwave, but not on the stove or in the oven? Is it safe to heat food up from the inside out, and how is the machine doing this? Why is the food heated unevenly? Is it good to heat your food that quickly?

Don't do it guys. Throw the microwave out, or drag it in the back yard and beat it with a baseball bat Office Space style. Just make sure you're playing Geto Boys "Damn It Feels Good To Be A Gangsta" in the background, and that you tape it and put it somewhere on social media and tag me! You'll live just fine without it, trust me…

High-Speed Fat Loss Guide

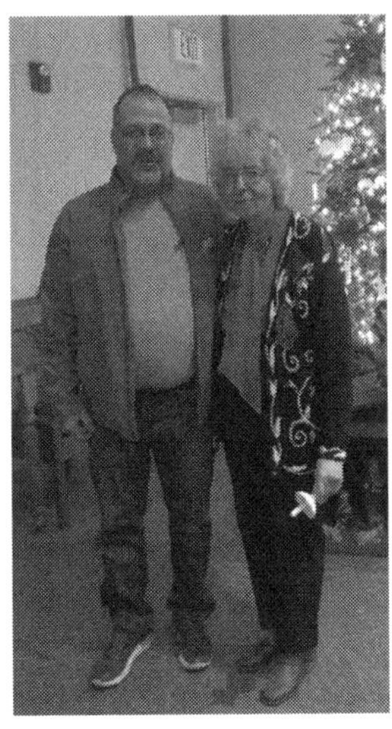

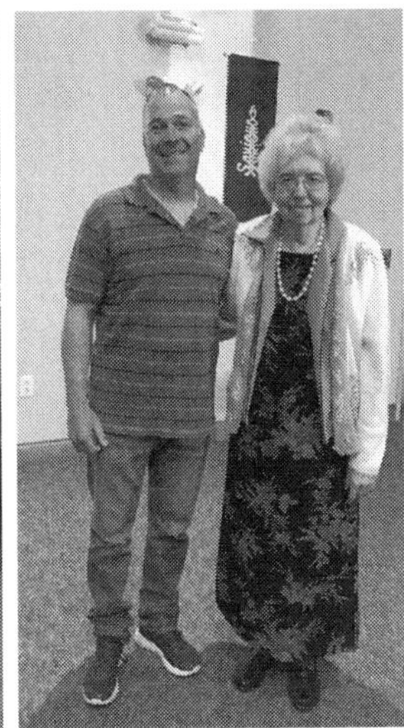

The high-speed fat loss guide (HSFL from now on) is the most challenging set of guidelines we have to offer. Challenging, but effective!

The man in the previous pictures is none other than Jonathan Martindale, my foreword contributor. Jonathan lost 55 pounds in just a little over 5 weeks, but are results like this typical? Absolutely! Even though this guide may be the most challenging, you still will not feel like you are on a diet due to the satiety the foods you will be eating provide.

There should also be no post weight loss binging or weight gain as long as you recycle the weeks as I will explain. During these three weeks, we strip the nutrients down to the bare bones which means we leave just enough to keep you alive!

Physiological effects we can expect are reduced weight, reduced fat, reduced energy in some cases depending on how addicted you have been to sugar (after the first 7-10 days), sweet cravings (after the first 7-10 days), a headache or two (between days 10-14), and if we are working out really hard, some lightheadedness.

Mentally, the HSFL guide is the hardest one to accomplish, but it will pay off big dividends in body fat reduction, hence the name. While some people may be more mentally strong than others, I do not recommend staying on this guide for more than 3 weeks. The physiological and psychological stress is too high, and we will burn out the adrenal glands. All of my guides are nutrient restrictive, not calorically restrictive, so eat as much as you can on the allowable food list to stay full and feel satisfied.

You will notice that the first week's list is not really that bad, but then you start to see things disappear more and more till you reach week three and it feels like you're only eating dry chicken and drinking water. On average people lose between 10-15 pounds in three weeks time, and one person even lost 21 pounds. One pound per day is completely safe and should be easy to accomplish. The crux of a good diet is two fold: one, it breaks bad habits for eating whatever you want, when you want, and two, when the weight goes it is gone forever! As extreme as this guide is, I have never had anyone lose 15 pounds, then gain 20 back, or even 10, or even 5! It's done methodically, and as long as we return to the maintenance diet after week three, you'll be fine and the weight loss should be permanent.

As a general rule of thumb, I have my clients use this guide for three weeks, then take one week where they eat from the maintenance guide. This stops your body from feeling like it is starving which causes it to be stingy when called upon to release fat from the cell. After the week on the maintenance guide you can go back to the HSFL guide for another three weeks. Repeat as necessary!

WEEK 1 ALLOWABLE FOODS

Breakfast:

Fat & Protein
Eggs
Bacon
Sausage
Hamburger Patties
Pork Belly
Ham
Grass Fed Butter

Carbs
Spinach
Cauliflower
Broccoli
Organic Celery
Asparagus
Mushrooms
Onions
Sauerkraut
Kimchi
Any and all herbs

Drinks
Coffee
Water
Unsweetened Nut Milk

Lunch and Dinner:

Any and all meats

Carbs
Avocado
Artichokes
Asparagus
Beans (must be heated)
Bean sprouts
Broccoli
Brussel sprouts
Cabbage
Cauliflower
Organic Celery
Daikon
Kale
Leeks
Mushrooms
Okra
Onions
Green Plantains
Radishes
Rutabaga
Salad greens (chicory, endive, escarole, iceberg lettuce, romaine, spinach, arugula, radicchio, watercress)
Shallots
Spinach
Swiss chard
Water chestnuts
Watercress

Any and all herbs

Drinks
Wine, water, unsweetened nut milk, Kombucha

Snacks

Raw macadamia nuts, walnuts, pecans, and pistachio nuts

Cheese, Goat Cheese
Prosciutto

Week 2 ALLOWABLE FOODS

Breakfast:

Fat & Protein
Eggs
Bacon
Pork Belly
Sausage
Grass Fed Butter

Carbs
Spinach
Cauliflower
Broccoli
Organic Celery
Asparagus
Mushrooms
Onions
Sauerkraut
Kimchi
Any and all herbs

Drinks
Coffee
Water
Unsweetened Nut Milk
Kombucha

Lunch and Dinner:

Red meat max for only 3 meals this week. Lamb, fish, and pork should be the remainder; one night of chicken is ok.

Carbs
Asparagus
Broccoli
Brussel sprouts
Cauliflower
Organic Celery
Cabbage (green, bok choy, Chinese)
Greens (collard, kale, mustard, turnip)
Kale
Leeks
Mushrooms
Okra
Onions
Radishes
Rutabaga
Salad greens (chicory, endive, escarole, iceberg lettuce, romaine, spinach, arugula, radicchio, watercress)
Spinach
Swiss chard
Any and all herbs

Drinks
Water, Unsweetened nut milk, Kombucha

Snacks
Raw macadamia nuts, walnuts, pecans and pistachio nuts

Goat cheese
Prosciutto

Week 3 ALLOWABLE FOODS

Breakfast:

Protein
Eggs
Ground turkey
Ground pork
Cook in:
Grass Fed Butter
Supplement:
Udo's Oil

Carbs
Asparagus
Broccoli
Cauliflower
Organic Celery
Mushrooms
Onions
Any and all herbs

Drinks
Coffee
Water
Unsweetened Nut Milk
Kombucha

Lunch and Dinner:

Protein: No Red Meat. Fish, turkey, or pork only

Carbs
Asparagus
Broccoli
Brussel sprouts
Cabbage (green, bok choy, Chinese)
Cauliflower
Organic Celery
Greens (collard, kale, mustard, turnip)
Kale
Mushrooms
Onions
Radishes
Salad greens (Kale, Arugula, Spinach)
Any and all herbs

Drinks
Water, Unsweetened nut milk, Kombucha

Snacks

Raw macadamia nuts, raw walnuts, pecans and raw pistachio nuts

Goat cheese
Prosciutto

Sample Day for Week 1:

Upon rising- make Bulletproof Coffee

When hunger begins (breakfast): Two hamburger patties with scrambled egg and avocado, plus a spoonful of Udo's oil.

When hunger begins again (lunch): Grass fed Ribeye steak, 4 organic celery stalks, and mushrooms to satiate, one bottle of Kombucha (always check the sugar content, then check the serving size. The good Kombucha's have 2-4 grams of sugar per serving, the bad have a whopping 16-20 per serving which gives you 32-40 grams of sugar per bottle which is a no-no)!

Snack or Pre work out: Handful of nuts with a or small coffee (only utilize if you are super duper hungry, remember the postprandial period!)

Dinner/Post Workout: Large cut of Salmon with lemon, kale, and boiled broccoli and cauliflower.

A spoonful of Udo's oil before bed. If you are over 200lbs. 2 spoonful's!

Notice I say, "When hunger begins." I have no pre-set time to start eating; only when I start to get hungry do I have something to eat. A lot of diets will tell you to eat at specific times, or eat 6 meals a day. On most days, I eat only two large meals. The other times that I eat I will snack on bacon, sausage, or hamburger patties, all fed an indigenous diet of course!

When people ask about snacks, they are thinking along the lines of protein bar, yogurt, chips, etc. Why not have a small hamburger with sauerkraut as a snack. Why does a snack have to come in a box or a bag and be made in a factory? On this guide, it is very important to eat as much natural, organic food as possible, and I would eat organic celery every day because it is a natural diuretic, and is actually one of the only foods that requires more calories to digest than it provides for the body. Again, never eat soft, limp celery because it contains a toxin you do not want to ingest!

Sample Week 1:

	Monday	Tuesday	Wednesday	Thursday	Friday	Saturday	Sunday
Breakfast	Bulletproof Coffee, or sausage w/sauerkraut	Bulletproof Coffee, or hamburger patties w/mushrooms	Bulletproof Coffee, or scrambled eggs, n bacon	Bulletproof Coffee, or pork belly, kimchi	Bulletproof Coffee, or omelet w/mushrooms, celery, spinach	Bulletproof Coffee, or hard boiled eggs, salted and peppered	Bulletproof Coffee, or ham steak, eggs, spinach & mushroom salad w/Udo's oil
Lunch	Skirt Steak with a raw salad, 1tsp Udo's oil	Lamb steak with an avocado 1tsp Udo's oil	Meatloaf w/arugula salad 1tsp Udo's oil	Rib eye steak w/ sautéed mushrooms, and navy beans 1tsp Udo's oil	Pork chops with steamed broccoli 1tsp Udo's oil	Ground beef w/ a salad, 1 tsp. Udo's oil	Lamb chops w/ boiled broccoli, cauliflower, celery 1tsp Udo's oil
Snack	Prosciutto, raw pistachio nuts	Hamburger patty	Two seasoned chicken thighs, Kombucha	Handful of raw walnuts, goat cheese	Spinach salad w/chopped nuts and goat cheese	Kombucha, prosciutto, raw macadamia nuts, goat cheese	½ cup seasoned ground beef topped w/ avocado
Dinner	Swordfish, w/ sautéed asparagus & Portabella mushrooms (supplement w/enzymes since there is no raw food) Apple cider vinegar shot	Mahi Mahi, spinach salad with beans, onions, tomatoes, artichokes Apple cider vinegar shot before bed	Chicken thighs w/ mushroom medley sprinkled with Udo's oil, Apple cider vinegar shot before bed	Turkey burgers w/avocado, and mashed cauliflower Apple cider vinegar shot before bed	Coconut shrimp with salad, Udo's oil, Apple cider vinegar shot before bed	Salmon w/ sautéed brussel sprouts, onions & asparagus Apple cider vinegar shot before bed	Seasoned duck breast w/ baked broccoli, artichoke, shallots, coconut oil, salt, pepper, Apple cider vinegar shot before bed

Sample Week 2:

	Monday	Tuesday	Wednesday	Thursday	Friday	Saturday	Sunday
Breakfast	Bulletproof Coffee, or scrambled eggs n bacon	Bulletproof Coffee, or sausage w/sauerkraut	Bulletproof Coffee, or pork belly, kimchi	Bulletproof Coffee, or omelet w/celery, spinach, mushroom, onions	Bulletproof Coffee, or sausage, mushrooms, onions	Bulletproof Coffee, or hard boiled eggs, kimchi	Bulletproof Coffee, or pork belly, sautéed spinach, onions
Lunch	Seasoned hamburger w/radishes, rutabaga 1tsp Udo's oil	Seasoned chicken thighs, steamed broccoli, cauliflower 1tsp Udo's oil	Ribeye steak, raw, celery, cooked bean salad 1tsp Udo's oil	Sashimi w/ sautéed asparagus, mushrooms, onions 1tsp Udo's oil	Ground turkey w/ peppers, leeks, tomatoes 1tsp Udo's oil	Porterhouse steak, raw spinach, onion, mushroom salad 1tsp Udo's oil	Duck breast w/ pinto beans, steamed brussel sprouts 1tsp Udo's oil
Snack	Kombucha, raw macadamia nuts	Goat cheese w/ raw pistachio's	Prosciutto, unsweetened coconut milk	Kombucha raw macadamia nuts	Prosciutto, raw pistachio nuts	Seasoned chicken thighs	Seasoned ground turkey
Dinner	Duck breast w/raw arugula mushroom, salad Apple cider vinegar shot before bed	Alaskan Salmon w/ raw organic celery stalks, steamed broccoli Apple cider vinegar shot before bed	Chicken Thighs steamed, mashed cauliflower Apple cider vinegar shot before bed	Pork loin sautéed asparagus, mushrooms, onions Apple cider vinegar shot before bed	Grass fed lamb chops w/ chopped macadamia nut lettuce salad Apple cider vinegar shot before bed	Steamed Halibut with asparagus Apple cider vinegar shot before bed	Pork chops w/ sautéed mushrooms, onions Apple cider vinegar shot before bed

Sample Week 3:

Week 3 is where things get tough. You're eating the same food, you don't have the same energy, in some cases you may have a headache from the lack of sugar you are no longer consuming, but this is where most of the magic happens. I call this the dry week. No alcohol, no sugar, no fun. Often times I'll eat the same vegetables for dinner that I did for lunch. You definitely want to take advantage of coffee this week, especially if you are exercising through all of this and do so later in the evening. I have coffee programmed in twice a day. The morning should be caffeinated, but you have the option in the evening to use decaf if you are sensitive to caffeine. What we are looking for is the hunger killing effect of caffeine that coffee has. This, in combination with being able to add healthy fats to the coffee, keeps us psychologically sound and blunt hunger while we lose fat at an alarming rate. If you don't have a blender at work, you can always add heavy whipping cream, or a generous amount of full fat canned coconut milk. Mixing the two together is an even better idea!

We are getting rid of all red meat for this week. Doing this greatly reduces our calories and this is how we start to lose the extra fat/weight. If you want to retain more muscle mass it is imperative that you lift heavy this week in all the classic lifts like the squat, deadlift, clean, snatch, and press. When I say heavy, I mean sets of 5-2 reps, no one reps maxes. Lifting heavy forces your body to retain your muscle. If you are not concerned with losing too much muscle, and are looking for more of an overall weight loss, then continue to lift and workout as normal. Lastly, make sure to eat plenty of fermented foods and have a shot of apple cider vinegar before you go to bed every night to keep the immune system strong!

Sample Week 3:

	Monday	Tuesday	Wednesday	Thursday	Friday	Saturday	Sunday
Breakfast	Bulletproof Coffee, or scrambled eggs w/mushrooms and onions 1 tsp. Udo's oil	Bulletproof Coffee, or two seasoned ground turkey patties 1 tsp. Udo's oil	Bulletproof Coffee, or hard boiled eggs, steamed broccoli and cauliflower 1 tsp. Udo's oil	Bulletproof Coffee, or two seasoned ground turkey patties, steamed asparagus 1 tsp. Udo's oil	Bulletproof Coffee, or ground pork w/sautéed onion, mushroom, celery 1 tsp. Udo's oil	Bulletproof Coffee, or scrambled eggs w/cheddar cheese 1 tsp. Udo's oil	Bulletproof Coffee, or ground chicken w/sautéed asparagus, mushrooms 1 tsp. Udo's oil
Lunch	Turkey breast w/ sautéed asparagus, mushrooms, onion	Pork loin w/ steamed broccoli, cabbage, cauliflower, Kombucha	Pasture raised Chicken thighs w sautéed yams	Baked fish, raw radishes, broccoli, cauliflower	Turkey patties w/ kale & arugula salad, Kombucha	Pork chops, spinach, raw mushroom salad	Pasture raised Chicken thighs, organic celery stalks
Snack	Bulletproof Coffee, raw walnuts, raw organic celery sticks	Bulletproof Coffee, raw pecans	Bulletproof Coffee, raw almonds, goat cheese	Bulletproof Coffee, raw macadamia nuts	Bulletproof Coffee, raw pistachio nuts, raw organic celery sticks	Bulletproof Coffee, raw pecans, goat cheese	Bulletproof Coffee, prosciutto

Dinner	Pork loin w/ mushrooms, onions, raw celery stalks, Apple cider vinegar shot, 1-3tsp of Udo's oil if you still feel hungry before bed	Salmon w/ grilled green plantains, Apple cider vinegar shot, 1-3tsp of Udo's oil if you still feel hungry before bed	Halibut w/sautéed brussel sprouts, mushrooms, Apple cider vinegar shot, 1-3tsp of Udo's oil if you still feel hungry before bed	Raw Ahi Tuna sautéed spinach, onion, asparagus, Apple cider vinegar shot, 1-3tsp of Udo's oil if you still feel hungry before bed	Salmon w/ cooked spinach, mushroom, pine nut salad, Apple cider vinegar shot, 1-3tsp of Udo's oil if you still feel hungry before bed	Pork chops w/ sautéed mushrooms, asparagus, brussel sprouts, Apple cider vinegar shot, 1-3tsp of Udo's oil if you still feel hungry before bed	Scallops on a bed of spinach & mushrooms, Apple cider vinegar shot, 1-3tsp of Udo's oil if you still feel hungry before bed

Maintenance Guide

The maintenance guide is geared towards just what it says, maintaining your bodyweight and fat index's. Its not geared toward performance, nor is it as mind bending as the High Speed Fat Loss guide, but rather a middle of the road, I just want to look good naked, or have enough energy to work out because its fun guide. The only thing we have to measure is our carbohydrate intake. We must stay between 100-120 grams of carbs a day. No more.

The maintenance guide is really just about balance. We want to eat more fat and protein in the morning with low glycemic carbohydrates. This ensures that we will keep burning fat for fuel after we wake up. You can have any type of meat at lunch that you desire. If I am a little more hungry than usual, I will eat my fattier types of meat like beef, pork, or chicken thighs instead of chicken breasts to keep me fuller for longer. It's usually nuts or goat cheese for a snack, then light protein (by light I mean the fat content and am talking about chicken breasts, fish or turkey) for dinner with my higher glycemic carbs to take advantage of our carb loading theory we talked about earlier. Don't worry; all of this will be spelled out in the allowable food list below.

Breakfast:

Fat & Protein
Eggs
Bacon
Beef
Cheese
Sausage
Hamburger Patties
Ham
Pork Belly
Grass Fed Butter

Carbs
Avocado
Cabbage (green, bok choy, Chinese)
Cauliflower
Kimchi
Salad greens (chicory, endive, escarole, iceberg lettuce, romaine, spinach, arugula, radicchio, watercress)
Sauerkraut
Spinach
Ezekiel Bread
Mana Bread
Any and all herbs

Lunch:
Any and all meats

Carbs
Asparagus
Avocado
Broccoli
Brussels sprouts
Cauliflower
Organic Celery
Cucumber
Daikon
Eggplant
Greens (collard, kale, mustard, turnip)
Kale
Leeks
Mushrooms
Onions
Okra
Radishes

Drinks
Water, nut milks with or without sugar

Snacks
Any and all raw nuts
Cheese
Beef jerky
Almond Butter
Cashew Butter
Coconut Butter
Prosciutto

Dinner:

Light protein – pasture raised chicken breasts, wild caught fish, and turkey

Carbs

Asparagus
Avocado
Mushrooms
Onions
Basmati rice
Bean sprouts
Broccoli
Brussel sprouts
Cabbage (green, bok choy, Chinese)
Cauliflower
Celery
Cucumber
Daikon
Kale
Leeks
Greens (collard, kale, mustard, turnip)
Okra
Radishes
Rutabaga
Salad greens (chicory, endive, escarole, iceberg lettuce, romaine, spinach, arugula, radicchio, watercress)
Spinach
Sugar snap peas
Swiss chard
Water chestnuts
Watercress
White Rice

Rye Bread
Sourdough Bread
Any and all herbs

Drinks

Beer, wine, water, and nut milks with or without sugar

Desserts

Coconut milk ice cream

Sample Day:

Eat 6-8 oz. of solid protein with every meal.

Meal one: Bacon and eggs, two slices of Ezekiel bread with butter, coffee with heavy cream or coconut milk.

Meal two: One pork chop with sautéed zucchini and mushrooms, a salad, and a couple scoops of almond, or coconut butter.

Snack (if you're training late): Handful of raw pecans, two slices of cheese.

Meal three: One pasture raised chicken breast with white rice and beans, glass of almond milk and three scoops of coconut ice cream (if you had a hard training day).

The maintenance guide has options. If you're really strict and you do not eat that much sugar, or any sugar at all for most of the week, I would suggest once every ten days doing a light refeed on sugar to make sure you don't start to dry out if you're training really hard. The other option is to have a small amount of sugar every other night to keep the storage tanks from getting too low. This guide is loosely based off of a ketogenic diet. I was competing in Brazilian Jiu-Jitsu, triathlons and marathons while on a ketogenic diet and fared pretty well. The problem became that after long periods with no sugar, my muscles started to dry up and I looked very stringy, almost skinny, and not well. In the off-season when I gained a couple pounds back, I was always told how much better I looked. The secret is that for every 4 grams of carbohydrates you ingest, your body needs to retain 1 gram of water in order to assimilate the energy. While training and competing for triathlons and marathons I was on a ketogenic diet eating less than 50 grams of carbs per day. One lucky day I stumbled upon John Kiefer's article on carb loading and decided to give it a shot. I tanked a whole pizza one night and woke up shredded! My muscles were hard and full, and I had an amazing amount of energy the next day. Not to mention I slept like a baby! So the lesson is that being too strict is actually counterproductive and not healthy. That is why we only do the High Speed Fat Loss guide for three weeks!

You can be happy and successful on this maintenance guide. It offers just the right amount of leeway and a large selection of food to where you don't feel like you're on a diet, and the foods are still wholesome and delicious.

Recipe Time!

I have never come up with an amazing meal myself before. I always see something in a magazine, online, or on TV that makes my mouth water and then I try to make it the best I can with my own spin on it. I really don't know when I started doing this, but I made mashed cauliflower one day that got amazing reviews with my friend's family. He said that their son would not eat cauliflower no matter what, but when I made the mashed cauliflower, he thought it was mashed potatoes and couldn't get enough of it!

I figured as an added bonus, I would include it here. Hope you enjoy it just as much!

- Boil an entire head of cauliflower until very soft, and then drain water.

- Add half a can of coconut milk and half a stick of grass fed unsalted butter and stir rigorously mashing everything together. Another option is to put all of this in a high-speed blender.

- Once mashed, add Himalayan sea salt and ground pepper to taste. If you have a food processor you can blend it to make it even creamier!

Don't overdue it with the coconut milk because you do not want it to be too watery. If anything, add less, mix it, and then add more if you need too. I really hope you enjoy it, drop me a line if you do!

Sample Maintenance Guide Week:

	Monday	Tuesday	Wednesday	Thursday	Friday	Saturday	Sunday
Breakfast	Bulletproof Coffee, or 3 eggs, bacon, sautéed spinach, mana bread	Bulletproof Coffee, or Pork Belly, sautéed mushrooms, onions	Bulletproof Coffee, or 2 eggs on top of 2 hamburger patties	Bulletproof Coffee, or sausage & cheese omelet, sauerkraut	Bulletproof Coffee, or steak & eggs, mana bread	Bulletproof Coffee, or omelet w/mushroom onions	Bulletproof Coffee, or pork belly, kimchi, mana bread
Lunch	Skirt steak salad, w/mushrooms, avocado, tomato	Ground beef with a raw arugula salad, with red peppers and chopped pecans	Pasture raised Chicken thighs, sautéed asparagus, Kombucha	Short ribs, sautéed collard greens, avocado	Hamburger patties, ketchup, mustard, on Ezekiel bread	Ribeye steak, mashed cauliflower, arugula salad	Pork chops, sautéed onions, spinach, kale
Snack	Raw pecans, goat cheese	Organic Celery stalks, macadamia nut butter	Macadamia nuts, beef jerky	Two scoops coconut butter, raw almonds	Raw walnuts, goat cheese,	Prosciutto, raw pistachios	Organic celery stalks, almond butter

Dinner	Duck breast, arugula salad w/ bean sprouts, cucumber, shot of apple cider vinegar before bed	Pork loin, basmati rice, snap peas, sourdough bread with butter, shot of apple cider vinegar before bed	Pasture raised Chicken thighs, steamed vegetable mix, shot of apple cider vinegar before bed	Salmon, asparagus, mushrooms, coconut milk ice cream shot of apple cider vinegar before bed	Lamb chops, asparagus, rye bread, shot of apple cider vinegar before bed	Sushi, coconut ice cream, shot of apple cider vinegar before bed	Wild caught halibut, mashed cauliflower, shot of apple cider vinegar before bed

Performance Guide

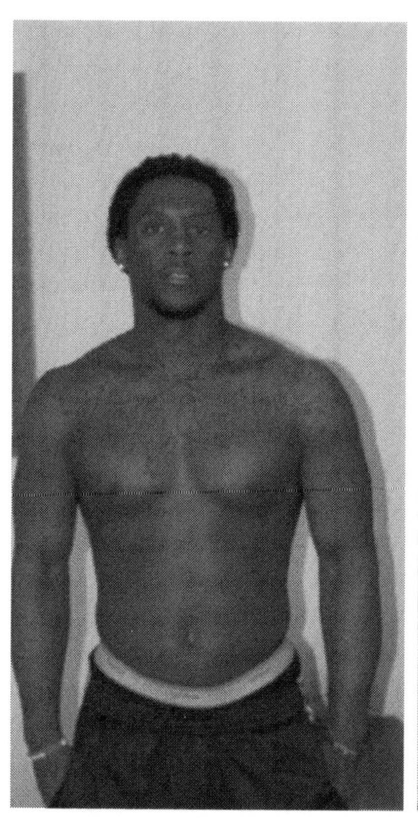

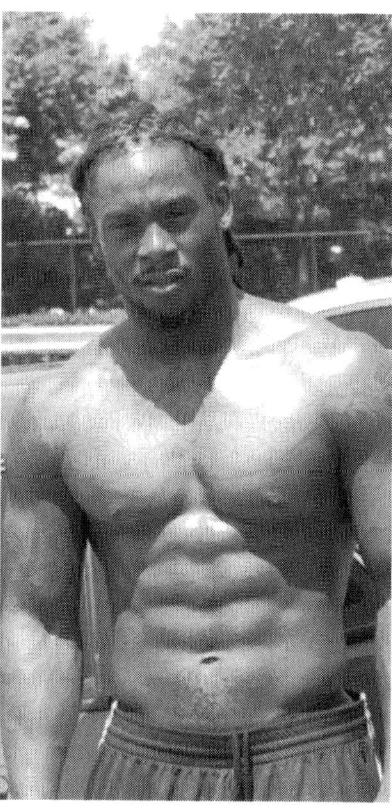

The performance guide is unlike anything you have ever tried. The athlete in the picture is Davone Bess, former wide receiver of the Miami Dolphins. Davone brought me down to Florida to work with him one on one after his second year in the NFL. The picture on the left is what he looked like on the first day I arrived in South Florida. The picture on the right was three months later when he was going into spring camp. Which one would you rather have on your team? The performance guide is based off of John Kiefer's carb loading program. The key physiological mechanisms were already discussed so I will not go into detail once again here. The basic premise is to train insane, and then eat a boatload of sugary carbohydrates in the evening time when your body is primed to use it for muscle growth and not for fat storage.

When I talk to people about carb loading I always reference their car or truck as an example. I ask them if they put gasoline in their car every day before they leave to go somewhere and they say of course not. I tell them that sugary carbs are meant to refill your energy stores once they are depleted. If you're eating them every day, even just a little piece of chocolate here and there, you are not using this guide correctly.

This guide can be utilized in two ways. If you are training to be a serious athlete, you will refeed multiple times per week. If you are just trying to look jacked and lean, and performance is not a serious issue, then I would carb load once every 5-7 days. The main point is to stay as carbohydrate (especially sugar) free all the way until you train. When you train, it needs to be heavy, and intense. Cardio, or going for a light jog does not constitute a carb load. When we sit down for dinner, you want to eat light protein (chicken, fish, turkey), and then as much sugar as possible. If you do it right, not only are you going to get the best night of sleep you have ever had in your entire life, but you will also wake up in a puddle of sweat; the reason being pretty fascinating actually.

You see, when we over consume calories, and the body has no place to put the extra, it then has to cook the extra calories off as heat by raising your body temperature. Me, as well as my athletes, have many great stories of waking up in the middle of the night and throwing the covers off feeling like a furnace! This all goes back to blocking the body's ability to put fat in the fat cell. Once the muscles are filled with fat and sugar, our metabolism will kick the heat up a couple notches and sweat the remainder of those calories out.

Another important aspect of this guide yields that you cannot eat anything for at least one hour after training. This is why it is ideal to train between 3:30pm and 5:30pm. If you train at 7:30pm, that means you wont finish till 8:30pm which means you should not eat till 9:30. That's a little late for most people. This is another one of John Kiefer's hacks. I used to be the guy preaching that a post workout shake should be consumed within 15 minutes of training. The weird thing was that no matter what I put in this post workout shake, it never felt like it was working.

Kiefer explains that exercise, to the body, is a catabolic process, meaning that it breaks things down. When we exercise we create a lot of disorder in the body and we kick in what is called the hermetic effects, or hormesis. **Hormesis** is a biological phenomenon whereby a beneficial effect (improved health, stress tolerance, growth or longevity) results from exposure to low doses of an agent that is otherwise toxic or lethal when given at higher doses. Exercise lethal? You betcha. There are many cases of rhabdomyolosis in CrossFit and Triathlons, as well as people dying running marathons. Small doses of exercise, (like the usual hour per day), break the body down slightly so it can regenerate to be bigger, faster, or stronger. It needs time to do this though and cannot be interrupted by the introduction of a post work out shake.

When you don't eat for an hour after exercise the immune system gets a chance to release cells called macrophage's to run around the body, scrape things down, and clean them up. When this process goes uninterrupted, you will recover much better. If you eat or have a shake directly after, this process gets neglected because the brain has to instruct the immune system to stay in the digestive tract in order to process the food. Ever since I started waiting one hour after training to introduce food, my recovery has been much better and I have been able to train harder. Before we get started with the food tables, lets list the major steps:

- No carbs, especially sugar before training.
- Train heavy and intense between 3:30pm and 5:30pm
- Wait 1 hour before eating any food, or having a post workout shake if you are on the road.
- Eat light protein and heavily sugared carbohydrates like donuts, pies, ice cream, cookies, etc. until you are full or content.

Some of you are saying, “But Chris, I train in the morning!” I hear you; I also train on most mornings. The protocol is still the same; we just will not get an **OPTIMAL** result, that’s all. I train most days between 9-11am. I eat a big lunch filled with meat and cruciferous vegetables, then I start to carb load after 5:30pm with cookies, coconut milk (the sugary kind in the carton) and the like all the way until I go to bed. Just to be on the safe side, I will write out two sample days for you; one where training occurs in the morning, and one where training occurs in the evening.

Sample carb loading day when training in the morning:

Upon Rising: Make bulletproof coffee.

Train at 10am

Lunch at Noon (Hormesis from 11-12): Two hamburgers, with sautéed mushrooms, salt and pepper. Avocado, and organic celery sticks.

Snack of raw walnuts, goat cheese

When hunger begins: Light protein like chicken fish or turkey. Cookies, apple pie, ice cream, donuts, and any type of sugary dessert you enjoy.

Before bed: Try to eat again if you can. Finish off that tub of ice cream; eat those donuts or cookies with coconut milk so they go down easier. Your goal should be to eat about 2000-5000 calories in carbohydrates before you go to bed.

Sample carb loading day when training in the afternoon:

Upon Rising: Make bulletproof coffee.

Lunch at Noon: Two hamburgers, with sautéed mushrooms, salt and pepper. Avocado, and organic celery sticks.

Train at 3-4 pm

Hormesis from 4-5, then

When hunger begins: Light protein like chicken fish or turkey. Cookies, apple pie, ice cream, donuts, and any type of sugary dessert you enjoy.

Before bed: Try to eat again if you can. Finish off that tub of ice cream; eat those donuts or cookies with coconut milk so they go down easier. Your goal should be to eat about 2000-5000 calories in carbohydrates before you go to bed.

ALLOWABLE FOODS

Breakfast:

Fat & Protein

Eggs
Bacon
Sausage
Hamburger Patties
Pork Belly
Ham
Grass Fed Butter

Carbs

Asparagus
Broccoli
Cauliflower
Kimchi
Mushrooms
Onions
Organic Celery
Sauerkraut
Spinach
Any and all herbs

Drinks

Coffee
Water
Nut Milk

Lunch and Dinner:

Any and all meats

Carbs

Avocado
Artichokes
Asparagus
Bean sprouts
Broccoli
Brussels sprouts
Cabbage
Cauliflower
Organic Celery
Cucumber
Daikon
Eggplant
Kale
Leeks
Mushrooms
Okra
Onions
Radishes
Rutabaga
Salad greens (chicory, endive, escarole, iceberg lettuce, romaine, spinach, arugula, radicchio, watercress)

Shallots
Spinach
Swiss chard
Tomato
Water chestnuts
Watercress
Any and all herbs

Drinks
Wine, water, nut milk, Kombucha

Snacks
Any and all raw nuts
Cheese, Goat Cheese
Prosciutto

Sample Week:

	Monday	Tuesday	Wednesday	Thursday	Friday	Saturday	Sunday
Breakfast	Bulletproof Coffee, pork belly	Bulletproof Coffee, two sausage	Bulletproof Coffee, 5 pieces of bacon	Bulletproof Coffee, 3 scrambled eggs	Bulletproof Coffee, ground beef w/mushrooms	Bulletproof Coffee, steak & eggs	Bulletproof Coffee, mushroom, onion omelet
Lunch	Two hamburgers, arugula salad, avocado	Ribeye steak, mashed cauliflower	Ground lamb, organic celery stalks, steamed broccoli	Ground beef, salad with Udo's oil, pine nuts, red peppers	Pork chops, w/asparagus, baked beans	Lamb steak, w/sautéed brussel sprouts	NY Strip steak, sautéed asparagus, mushrooms
Snack	Prosciutto, Kombucha	Celery stalks w/coconut butter	Raw macadamia nuts, w/ goat cheese	Raw walnuts w/goat cheese	Prosciutto	Raw pecans out of the shell	Prosciutto, raw pistachios
Training Time	4:30	4:30	4:30	Day off	4:30	4:30	Day off

Dinner	2 chicken thighs, cookies, donuts, almond milk, enzymes	Sushi, apple pie, coconut ice cream, almond milk, enzymes	1 chicken breast, 2 bite brownies, box of cookies, lemonade, enzymes	Halibut, mashed cauliflower, arugula salad, enzymes	Tuna, pint of cashew ice cream, cookies, enzymes	1 chicken breast, banana cream pie, almond milk, enzymes	Pork loin, steamed broccoli, zucchini, enzymes

As you can see, on the days we do not train, we eat a lower amount of carbohydrates throughout the whole day. Just because the day calls for a carb load does not necessarily mean we have to do one either. I have had plenty of athletes train very hard, go home and sit in front of a tub of ice cream and have it not appeal to them. This is your body telling you something so listen to it! Some days it may say eat everything and the kitchen sink, and some days it may say just have a few cookies and you're good. If I ever start to feel bloated or weighed down by the grains and junk food, I eat clean for two days in a row, maybe three, my system clears, and I feel much better. One of my favorite aspects of this guide is that it eliminates the need for a protein shake after the workout. You wait an hour after training, then the gloves come off and you eat whatever you want. Post workout nutrition has evolved to say the least! I laugh when I see diet plans in the magazines calling for you to weigh your food and eat nothing but chicken and mixed vegetables in order to get lean. Anyone can starve him or herself and lose weight, but can you feel good and lose fat? I don't think so, I know so.

This guide does so many things on so many levels it really is somewhat the best way to eat. Kiefer says EVERYONE should eat his or her carbs in the evening and I tend to believe him. This guide works on the physiological and psychological level at the same time. With food, willpower works for only so long, and in some cases not at all. The wrong types of food can actually change the chemistry in your brain, which changes the signals your body sends to the brain, ultimately changing your cravings. It doesn't matter how much willpower you have, because you are no longer in control. Your brain is sending the cravings automatically, and once we get to this point we are in major trouble nutritionally.

A couple of final points to make here is to use high amounts of discretion when utilizing the carb loading aspect of this diet. This does not mean we get to load up on the nastiest processed food we can find. My carb loads these days are done with a lot of coconut ice cream and gluten free cookies. Some junk is thrown in there every once in awhile but for the most part I still try to eat as clean as possible when I carb load. One of the main things we have to be careful of when we are carb loading is food coloring. Food coloring these days is being closely linked to many different diseases. Here is a short, yet nasty list found on thetruthaboutcancer.com:

Blue #1 (Brilliant Blue) – found primarily in baked goods, beverages, and cereals. It caused kidney tumors in laboratory mice.

Blue #2 (Indigo Carmine) – colorant in candies, pet food, and other items. Shown to cause brain tumors in rats.

Green #3 (Fast Green) – found in many cosmetics, candy, and drugs. Increases tumors of the bladder and testes in male rats.

Red #3 (Erythrosine) – colors maraschino cherries, baked goods, and candy. Banned by the FDA for causing thyroid tumors when used in externally applied cosmetics and topical drugs.

Red #40 (Allura Red) – the most widely used dye found in cereals, desserts, drugs, and cosmetics. Accelerates immune system tumors in mice and triggers allergic reactions and hyperactivity in children.

Yellow #5 (Tartrazine) – found in any number of baked goods, cereal, gelatin products, and dessert powders. Causes severe hypersensitivity and triggers hyperactivity disorders and other behavioral issues in children.

Yellow #6 (Sunset Yellow) – Used in beverages, desserts, gelatin, candy, and even sausage. Found to cause adrenal tumors and trigger severe hyperactivity in children.

Reading that list makes me think twice about eating any type of artificially colored processed food. The sad fact is that children are the ones eating most of the artificial food coloring in their cereals, sports drinks that allegedly hydrate you, and candy these days. The super sad fact is that every color we need to make food look more appetizing can readily be made from natural sources. The European Union has been doing this for years now and has gone completely chemical and dye free.

Lastly, try to limit the amount of lecithin, and gums you are consuming, and I'm not talking bubble gum. I'm talking about guar gum and locust bean gum and whatever other food additives these scientist come up with. Gums are thickeners for milk, desserts, and used as a binding agent for meat. Even though they have been around since the 80's, there have been some unfortunate incidents with their assimilation in the human body, specifically guar gum. Guar gum can actively suppress appetite and regulate insulin and when manufacturers found this out, they created a weight loss pill from it. Unfortunately the pill was swelling and obstructing the esophagus and intestines of some of the users hospitalizing 10 people and killing one. Doctors believe the swelling and death were a result of a lack of fluids in their body, and in light of this the FDA pulled the product from the shelves deeming it unsafe.

Guar gum can also reduce the absorbability of dietary minerals in the very food you are consuming and in 2007 the

European commission issued a warning that high levels of dioxins (read really bad toxins) are found in guar gum as well. Finally, a small amount of soy protein is contained in guar gum as a result of the manufacturing process as well so those who have an allergy to soy make have a negative reaction after consuming it and be completely mystified as to why their favorite cake is making them break out. While you don't have to avoids gums like the plague, if you are carb loading more than once a week, you may start to build up more in your body than you would like so just make sure you are tracking your consumption of it. Awareness is the key to our health!

When it comes to lecithins our primary concern is once again the avoidance of soy. Lecithin is an emulsifier, which means it helps the ingredients in food mix and bind in a more suitable manor. Sunflower lecithin seems to be ok, but like I talked about in the protein section, soy is not a great substitute for dairy on any level, and men, women and children of all ages should be very wary of its consumption, or at least limit it to once or twice a month if you just can't let it go.

That brings the performance guide section to a close. While it seems that I am contradicting myself by telling you to avoid sugar and processed food, and then consume it for performance, it comes down to knowledge. We know what we have to do before we eat it (lift heavy), we know when we can consume it (in the evening time), and we know what to stay away from when we consume large amounts of sweets (food coloring, gums, lecithins, and high fructose corn syrup). If you have any further questions or want to do some more light reading on the subject, I highly suggest looking up John Kiefer's website www.body.io as there is lots of great information on there, and his podcasts are always a great listen as well!

Know Your Worth

The mini series Band of Brothers is one of my all time favorites. In part three, and episode called Carentan, Easy Company has to attack a town heavily occupied by German troops. They're successful in their attack, and just when they get a chance to rest, they find out more Germans are coming so they head out to meet them. There's a quick firefight as they each meet up with a massive field in between them and as night falls and the rain comes, fighting ceases for the moment. A private from another company left his foxhole alone to go to the bathroom and happened to stumble upon a Lieutenant Ronald Spears from D Company. Spears was already a legend in most of the men's eyes, pulling some pretty heroic stunts in the line of fire. The young private asked in admiration if Lieutenant spears was scared and what Spears said has stuck with me since this day. He said "The sooner you realize that you're already dead you'll be able to function how a soldier *should* function; with no remorse, regret, or hesitation." The young soldier was in complete shock because it wasn't the answer he was expecting, but Spears was right.

Most people go to war hoping they live through it. As Spears denied his fear of death, it allowed him to live more tenaciously. He was living with the end in mind, which allowed him to think faster and move through reflex rather than hesitation. When it comes to your nutrition I too want you to live with the end in mind and that end is ultimately how do you want to die? I would like to die healthy, not from disease. I would like to pass away in my sleep in my warm comfortable bed, not with tubes hanging out of me in the intensive care unit. I would like to have amazing experiences in my 70's and 80's, not wither away in an old folks home. I'm sure looking ahead you would like to die healthy as well, but are you making decisions in your daily life that reflect that? I hope after reading the last 216 pages you are starting to.

There are many facts presented in this book, not because they have been studied and peer reviewed, but because they have been lived *through* for very many years now and found to be true. Eat processed food, get sick. Eat sugar, get fat. Combine them both, get diabetes, heart disease, a fatty liver and a whole host of other debilitating diseases.

Other truths can be eat meat, get lean. Eat plants, reverse aging. Eat coconut oil, get energy. And there it is. The sad fact that most of the American public is not aware of is that corporations are not just selling you products, they are selling you addictions. You see, food is no longer the creation of God, or nature, it is now the creation of mankind. Food used to be limited, scarce even. Now it is limitless. We used to have to expend just as much energy hunting for and gathering it, as it would provide. Now, we can literally have it brought to our doorstep.

There is no protector of the universe when it comes to food. Our animal counterparts (unless being fed by humans) seem to know what's good for them, so why don't we?

As we established in the introduction, our nutrition these days is like a game of Ping-Pong between over observation, and misdirection. Of the thousands and thousands of studies done on the causation of heart disease, the truth of the matter is still up for debate. This is why there are just a little over 20 resources contained in this book. I only cite the material that I found to be true through my own use of food. With "research" studies being conducted by scientists who are paid to find a favorable result the company can campaign with, there is no one left to trust anymore except your own gut.

Use this guide deliberately and it will NOT fail you. Use it liberally and it may or may not work. Can you switch coffee to tea? Sure. I just don't KNOW if that will work as well. When it comes to nutrition, especially losing weight everyone wants to know what he or she can get away with and the answer is NOTHING. You either eat healthy and die healthy or eat poorly, and die sickly. I don't think you deserve that. I don't even know you but I believe you deserve better than that because I believe people are worth more than a stock price or bottom line. I believe you have a purpose in this world that may be getting masked by poor food choices. The greatest gift we can give to others and the world is more of ourselves and you can't do that if you die early. I don't care how much you love ding-dongs they're toxic and will take you from your friends and family well before your mission here on Earth is complete. In closing, I'd like to leave you with this quote:

"As long as you have certain desires about how it ought to be, you can't see how it is." -Ram Dass

Don't let these company's take more time and money from you than they already have. Eat real food and discover that proper nutrition isn't a diet – it's a lifestyle.

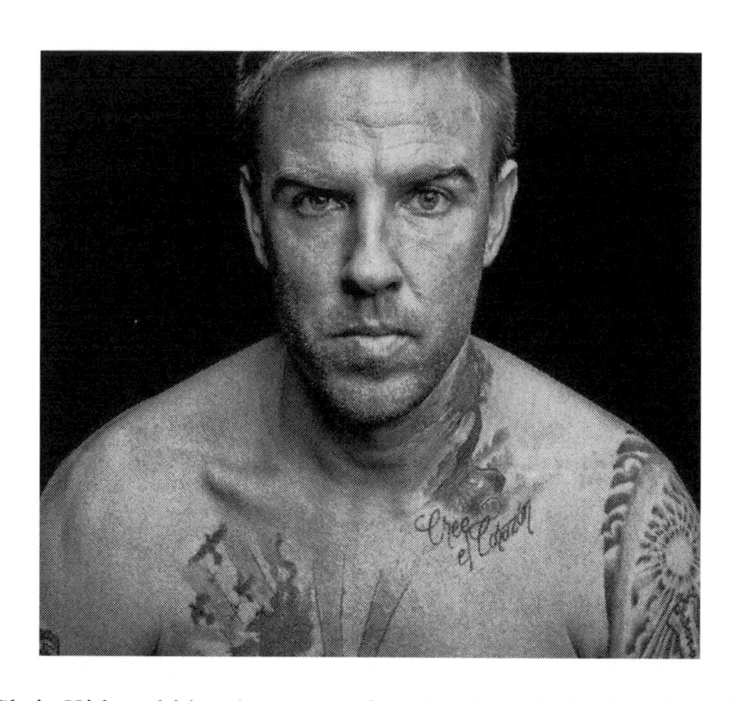

Chris Kidawski has been transforming lives in the health and fitness profession for the last 18 years. Armed with his master's in Kinesiology from the University of Hawai'i he helps heal and reverse disease from the inside out. Chris has trained people in all walks of life including but not limited to Navy SEALs, professional athletes, World Champion mixed martial artists, mothers, fathers, sons, daughters, and people just like you!

Chris has dedicated himself to discovering the truth about all aspects of health and wellness and has become as complete of a life coach as you can get. He has written two books so far, The Death Of Dieting which teaches you how to detoxify your body with natural, wholesome food, and The Everspace which teaches you how to operate from a place of stillness to achieve success in your life.

Chris now lives and runs his business Influential Health Solutions from sunny South Florida, but also does public speaking engagements and seminars in Universities, Corporations and gyms all over the country. He has been featured on many podcasts where he dives deeper into his body/spirit/mind paradigm of human health and thoroughly enjoys opening up people's lives with his information. For speaking engagements or to work with Chris email c.kidawski@gmail.com.

References

1. Colpo, Anthony. The Great Cholesterol Con: Why Everything You've Been Told about Cholesterol, Diet, and Heart Disease Is Wrong. Lulu.com, (2006) 426pp.

2. Erasmus, Udo. Fats that Heal, Fats that Kill. Alive Books, (1993) 456pp.

3. Miriam Goebel-Stengel,Tobias Hofmann,Ulf Elbelt,Pauline Teuffel,Anne Ahnis,Peter Kobelt,Nils W.G. Lambrecht,Burghard F. Klapp,Andreas Stengel. Peptides: The ghrelin activating enzyme ghrelin-O-acyltransferase (GOAT) is present in human plasma and expressed dependent on body mass index. Elsevier. Volume 43. May: 2013. PP 13-19.

4. McDougall, John. Marketing Milk and Disease. www.notmilk.com

5. Champ, Colin E. M.D. Misguided Medicine: The Truth Behind Ill Advised Medical Recommendations and How to Take Health Back Into Your Hands. CDR Health and Nutrition, LLC. 2014.

6. Kiefer, John. The Carb Nite Solution. Kiefer Productions, LLC. 2005.

7. http://www.barleymagic.com/enzymes.html

8. Greenfield, Ben. Beyond Training: Mastering Endurance, Health, and Life. Victory Belt Publishing, Inc. 2014.

9. Robert Dubrow, Amy S. Darefsky, Yikyung Park, Susan T. Mayne, Steven C. Moore, Briseis Kilfoy,

Amanda J. Cross, Rashmi Sinha, Albert R. Hollenbeck, Arthur Schatzkin, and Mary H. Ward. Dietary Components Related to *N*-Nitroso Compound Formation: A Prospective Study of Adult Glioma. Cancer Epidemiol Biomarkers Prev July 2010 19:1709-1722; Published OnlineFirst June 22, 2010; doi:10.1158/1055-9965.EPI-10-0225

10. Annie N. Samraj, Oliver M. T. Pearce, Heinz Laubli, Alyssa N. Crittenden, Anne K. Bergfeld, Kalyan Banda, Christopher J. Gregg, Andrea E. Bingman, Patrick Secrest, Nissi M. Varki, Ajit Varki. A red meat-derived glycan promotes inflammation and cancer progression. PNAS January 13, 2015 vol. 112 no. 2

11. Rawlings, Deirdre Ph.D., N.D. Fermented Foods for Health: Use the Power of Probiotic Foods to Improve Your Digestion, Strengthen Your Immunity, and Prevent Illness. Fair Winds Press, Beverly, Massachusetts.

12. Asprey, D. (2014). *The bulletproof diet: lose up to a pound a day, reclaim your energy and focus, and upgrade your life*. Emmaus, PA: Rodale Books.

13. http://articles.mercola.com/sites/articles/archive/2010/09/11/alkaline-water-interview.aspx

14. Chun Z. Yang, Stuart I. Yaniger, V. Craig Jordan, Daniel J. Klein, George D. Bittner Most Plastic Products Release Estrogenic Chemicals: A Potential Health Problem That Can Be Solved Environ Health Perspect. 2011 Jul 1; 119(7): 989–996. Published online 2011 Mar 2. doi: 10.1289/ehp.1003220

15. Gundry, S. R., & Buehl, O. B. (2017). *The plant paradox: the hidden dangers in "healthy" foods that cause disease and weight gain*. New York, NY: Harper Wave, an imprint of HarperCollins.
16. https://jonbarron.org/heart-health/can-cholesterol-go-too-low#
17. Mercola, J. (2017). *Fat for fuel: a revolutionary diet to combat cancer, boost brain power, and increase your energy*. Carlsbad, CA: Hay House, Inc.
18. Lane, N. (2009). *Power, sex, suicide: mitochondria and the meaning of life*. Oxford: Oxford University Press.
19. Avena, N. M., Rada, P., & Hoebel, B. G. (2009). Sugar and Fat Bingeing Have Notable Differences in Addictive-like Behavior. *The Journal of Nutrition*, *139*(3), 623–628. http://doi.org/10.3945/jn.108.097584.
20. Gersch et al. 2007. Fructose, but not dextrose, accelerates the progression of chronic kidney disease. American Journal of Physiology. Renal Physiology 293 (4): F1256-F1261.
21. Greger, M., & Stone, G. (2017). *How not to die: discover the foods scientifically proven to prevent and reverse disease*. London: Pan Books.
22. *JAMA Intern Med.* 2016;176(11):1680-1685. doi:10.1001/jamainternmed.2016.5394

Made in the USA
Middletown, DE
19 January 2018